Acute and Chronic Heart Failure: Pathophysiology and New Therapeutic Developments

Guest Editors

Serafino Fazio
Valentina Mercurio

MDPI

Basel • Beijing • Wuhan • Barcelona • Belgrade • Novi Sad • Cluj • Manchester

Guest Editors
Serafino Fazio
Department of Internal Medicine
Federico II University
Naples
Italy

Valentina Mercurio
Department of Translational Medical Sciences
Federico II University
Naples
Italy

Editorial Office
MDPI AG
Grosspeteranlage 5
4052 Basel, Switzerland

This is a reprint of the Special Issue, published open access by the journal *Biomedicines* (ISSN 2227-9059), freely accessible at: https://www.mdpi.com/journal/biomedicines/special_issues/WNSJL4DAS5.

For citation purposes, cite each article independently as indicated on the article page online and as indicated below:

Lastname, A.A.; Lastname, B.B. Article Title. *Journal Name* **Year**, *Volume Number*, Page Range.

ISBN 978-3-7258-5231-4 (Hbk)
ISBN 978-3-7258-5232-1 (PDF)
https://doi.org/10.3390/books978-3-7258-5232-1

Contents

About the Editors

Serafino Fazio

Serafino Fazio MD was born in Naples (ITALY) on February 5,1950. He received his scientific high school diploma June 1968. He received his master's degree in Medicine and Surgery at the University Federico II of Naples, School of Medicine on December 21, 1974. He specialized in Internal Medicine and in Cardiology. He is the author of more than 185 papers published on prestigious Journals. Among them are the *New England Journal of Medicine, Nature medicine, Annals of Internal Medicine, Circulation, International Journal of Cardiology, Biomedicines,* etc. He has been particularly interested in the interaction between hormones and the heart, heart failure treatment, Insulin resistance, metabolic syndrome, nutraceutical substances and, recently, Covid19 treatment. His h-hindex, according to Google scholar, is 48.

Valentina Mercurio

Valentina Mercurio is currently a tenure-track Assistant Professor of Medicine at Federico II University of Naples, Italy. She graduated in Medicine at the University of Naples Federico II, where she also completed her Fellowship in Internal Medicine and her PhD in Clinical and Experimental Medicine. She has also pursued advanced research training as a postdoctoral fellow at Johns Hopkins University in Baltimore, USA, further expanding her expertise. Her professional interests lie in chronic heart failure, pulmonary hypertension, and echocardiographic assessments of the right heart, with a commitment to integrating innovative approaches into clinical practice. Dr. Mercurio has been involved in several research projects, clinical trials, and academic publications, contributing to the growing body of knowledge in these fields. In addition to her clinical and research activities, Dr. Mercurio is passionate about medical education and actively participates in the training and mentoring of medical students and residents. She is also engaged in national and international scientific societies, reflecting her dedication to fostering a broader impact on healthcare delivery and patient outcomes.

biomedicines

MDPI

Editorial

Insulin Resistance with Associated Hyperinsulinemia as a Cause of the Development and Worsening of Heart Failure

Umberto Attanasio [1], Valentina Mercurio [1] and Serafino Fazio [2,*]

1 Department of Translational Medical Sciences, Federico II University, 80131 Naples, Italy; umberto.attanasio@yahoo.it (U.A.); valemercurio@yahoo.com (V.M.)
2 Department of Internal Medicine, School of Medicine, Federico II University, 80131 Naples, Italy
* Correspondence: fazio0502@gmail.com

Despite the considerable progress that has been made with regard to the prevention and treatment of cardiovascular diseases, heart failure (HF) remains a particularly important cause of recurring hospitalizations, with relevant social and healthcare costs, and it is a significant cause of mortality; as such, there is a need for continuous efforts to improve our understanding of its complex pathophysiology and refine relevant therapeutic strategies [1]. The incidence of HF, particularly HF with preserved ejection fraction (HFpEF), continues to rise, partly due to the increased prevalence of insulin resistance (IR) and the subsequent development of type 2 diabetes [2]. This Special Issue helps to shed light on various aspects of HF, with a notable focus on IR's role in its pathogenesis and the potential benefits of targeting IR to improve HF management.

Researchers are placing increasing emphasis on the intricate interplay between metabolic dysregulation and cardiac function. IR, which is characterized by impaired glucose uptake and utilization by cells, is often accompanied by hyperinsulinemia, a compensatory response aimed at maintaining glucose homeostasis [3,4]. While hyperinsulinemia initially helps regulate blood sugar levels, chronic elevation of insulin exerts detrimental effects on the cardiovascular system, ultimately contributing to HF progression [2]. Several mechanisms appear to link IR/hyperinsulinemia to HF. These include endothelial dysfunction, since IR is thought to interfere in the balance of vasodilating and vasoconstricting factors, leading to impaired endothelial function and increased vascular resistance [3]; left ventricular hypertrophy and remodeling, given that hyperinsulinemia promotes the proliferation of vascular smooth muscle cells and myocardiocytes, resulting in increased left ventricular mass and concentric remodeling (both hallmarks of HFpEF) [4]; myocardial lipid accumulation, occurring as a result of IR-related excess lipid deposition in the myocardium, which interferes with cell signaling and disrupts cardiac structure, leading to lipotoxicity and impaired heart function; and altered myocardial substrate metabolism, since IR shifts myocardial substrate utilization from glucose to free fatty acids, leading to metabolic inflexibility and reduced cardiac function. Furthermore, the association between serum free fatty acid levels and clinical parameters in acute HF patients highlights the complex metabolic dysregulation associated with acute HF, which is often characterized by increased reliance on fatty acid oxidation as an energy source due to impaired glucose utilization [5].

Despite these advances in knowledge, there are still significant gaps in our understanding of IR's precise role in the various HF subtypes and the optimal strategies for mitigating its adverse effects. This Special Issue addresses some of these gaps by exploring the impact of IR on different aspects of HF pathophysiology and investigating potential therapeutic targets.

The articles published in this Special Issue also offer new potential alternatives for clinical interventions, such as the possible use of point-of-care urine chloride measurement using strip tests as a tool to monitor fluid status and decongestive therapy in patients with HF. Furthermore, the potential therapeutic benefits of targeting IR in HF are explored. The review article discusses the negative impact of IR/hyperinsulinemia on chronic HF and proposes implementing early screening and treatment of IR to improve patient outcomes. The evidence suggests that substances such as metformin and berberine, which are known to reduce IR, may have clinical benefits for HF patients, while others, such as SGLT2 inhibitors and GLP-1 RA, have already proven their value in clinical settings [2]. These findings underscore the importance of considering IR as a modifiable risk factor and therapeutic target in HF management. While the articles in this Special Issue provide valuable contributions to the field, further research is needed to advance our understanding and management of IR in HF. Indeed, future studies should aim to elucidate the specific mechanisms by which IR contributes to the development and progression of various HF subtypes. This will enable the development of tailored therapeutic strategies based on the underlying pathophysiology. Studies should also focus on developing accurate and accessible methods for early IR screening in at-risk individuals and HF patients. Additionally, research is needed to determine the most effective therapeutic agents and optimal dosages for targeting IR in HF, considering potential drug interactions and patient-specific factors. Furthermore, assessing the effectiveness of different dietary approaches, exercise regimens, and combinations of lifestyle interventions in reducing IR and enhancing cardiac function may also provide some valuable information related to preventive medicine. Finally, efforts should focus on identifying and validating new therapeutic targets that specifically address the detrimental effects of IR on the cardiovascular system, with the aim of modulating insulin signaling pathways and improving metabolic flexibility in HF patients.

Conflicts of Interest: The authors declare no conflict of interest.

References

1. Ponikowski, P.; Voors, A.A.; Anker, S.D.; Bueno, H.; Cleland, J.G.F.; Coats, A.J.S.; Falk, V.; González-Juanatey, J.R.; Harjola, V.; Jankowska, E.A.; et al. 2016 ESC Guidelines for the diagnosis and treatment of acute and chronic heart failure. *Eur. J. Heart Fail.* **2016**, *18*, 891–975. [CrossRef] [PubMed]
2. Fazio, S.; Mercurio, V.; Affuso, F.; Bellavite, P. The Negative Impact of Insulin Resistance/Hyperinsulinemia on Chronic Heart Failure and the Potential Benefits of Its Screening and Treatment. *Biomedicines* **2023**, *11*, 2928. [CrossRef] [PubMed]
3. Mercurio, V.; Carlomagno, G.; Fazio, V.; Fazio, S. Insulin resistance: Is it time for primary prevention? *World J. Cardiol.* **2012**, *4*, 1–7. [CrossRef] [PubMed]
4. Freeman, A.M.; Acevedo, L.A.; Pennings, N. Insulin Resistance. 2023 Aug 17. In *StatPearls*; StatPearls Publishing: Treasure Island, FL, USA, 2024. [PubMed]
5. Klobučar, I.; Hinteregger, H.; Lechleitner, M.; Trbušić, M.; Pregartner, G.; Berghold, A.; Sattler, W.; Frank, S.; Degoricija, V. Association between Serum Free Fatty Acids and Clinical and Laboratory Parameters in Acute Heart Failure Patients. *Biomedicines* **2023**, *11*, 3197. [CrossRef] [PubMed]

biomedicines

Article

Role of Pericytes in Cardiomyopathy-Associated Myocardial Infarction Revealed by Multiple Single-Cell Sequencing Analysis

Yanqiao Lu †, Huanhuan Huo †, Feng Liang, Jieyuan Xue, Liang Fang, Yutong Miao, Lan Shen * and Ben He *

Department of Cardiology, Shanghai Chest Hospital, School of Medicine, Shanghai Jiao Tong University, Shanghai 200030, China; luyanqiao2013@live.com (Y.L.); huohuanhuan540@126.com (H.H.); liangfengwind@sjtu.edu.cn (F.L.); jieyuanxue@outlook.com (J.X.); fangliang0@foxmail.com (L.F.); miaoyutong8128@163.com (Y.M.)

* Correspondence: shenlan_shanghai@163.com (L.S.); heben241@126.com (B.H.)

† These authors contributed equally to this work.

Abstract: Acute myocardial infarction (AMI) is one of the leading causes of cardiovascular death worldwide. AMI with cardiomyopathy is accompanied by a poor long-term prognosis. However, limited studies have focused on the mechanism of cardiomyopathy associated with AMI. Pericytes are important to the microvascular function in the heart, yet little attention has been paid to their function in myocardial infarction until now. In this study, we integrated single-cell data from individuals with cardiomyopathy and myocardial infarction (MI) GWAS data to reveal the potential function of pericytes in cardiomyopathy-associated MI. We found that pericytes were concentrated in the left atrium and left ventricle tissues. *DLC1/GUCY1A2/EGFLAM* were the top three uniquely expressed genes in pericytes ($p < 0.05$). The marker genes of pericytes were enriched in renin secretion, vascular smooth muscle contraction, gap junction, purine metabolism, and diabetic cardiomyopathy pathways ($p < 0.05$). Among these pathways, the renin secretion and purine metabolism pathways were also found in the process of MI. In cardiomyopathy patients, the biosynthesis of collagen, modulating enzymes, and collagen formation were uniquely negatively regulated in pericytes compared to other cell types ($p < 0.05$). *COL4A2/COL4A1/SMAD3* were the hub genes in pericyte function involved in cardiomyopathy and AMI. In conclusion, this study provides new evidence about the importance of pericytes in the pathogenesis of cardiomyopathy-associated MI. *DLC1/GUCY1A2/EGFLAM* were highly expressed in pericytes. The hub genes *COL4A2/COL4A1/SMAD3* may be potential research targets for cardiomyopathy-associated MI.

Keywords: cardiomyopathy; myocardial infarction; pericytes; *SMAD3*

1. Introduction

Cardiovascular disease (CVD) is one of the leading causes of death worldwide, accounting for over 4 million deaths in Europe each year [1]. Acute myocardial infarction (AMI) is a life-threatening type of CVD that can cause malignant arrhythmia and sudden cardiac death [2]. When an artery becomes acutely blocked, blood flow is disrupted and the heart is unable to supply blood normally. Severe myocardial ischemia and hypoxia result in the damage and death of myocardial cells [3]. After the acute phase, adverse ventricular remodeling reduces cardiac function, resulting in heart failure and increased mortality [4]. In developed countries, AMI is one of the leading causes of death [5]. Despite rapid advances in therapeutic technology and out-of-hospital management [6], morbidity and mortality rates remain around 5% [7]. AMI with cardiomyopathy is a specific type of AMI. It is reported that patients with AMI and cardiomyopathy experience poorer long-term outcomes [8]. Few studies focus on the pathogenesis of AMI with cardiomyopathy. Most pathogenesis studies focus on the whole heart or major cell types in the heart, such as cardiomyocytes and macrophages [9–11]. The role of other cells in the pathogenesis of AMI with cardiomyopathy has not been well studied.

Microvascular pericytes and the recently discovered adventitial pericyte-like progenitors are closely associated with small and large vessels, respectively [12]. The role of pericytes in cardiovascular diseases has been increasingly recognized. Firstly, pericytes are a safe cell type. Furthermore, vascular pericytes are more abundant than other types of cells in the heart [13]. Pericyte dysfunction, on the other hand, may be involved in the pathogenesis of CVD [14], such as the processes involved in the regulation of cardiac homeostasis, angiogenesis, blood flow regulation, coagulation process regulation, and so on. Pericytes have received increasing attention for their applications in cardiovascular diseases, due to their pleiotropic and powerful angiogenic capacities [15]. The multipotent pericytes in capillaries are EphA7-positive, with angiogenic abilities [16]. During the progress of AMI, cardiac pericytes can migrate to the infarction zone and engage in the remodeling of the injured heart [17]. Cardiac pericytes upregulate the fibrosis-associated genes and matrix synthetic profiles, which promote the maturation of infarct vasculature in AMI [18]. Thus, understanding the crucial roles of pericytes in AMI may be helpful in identifying potential therapy targets for AMI.

In this study, we integrated single-cell RNA-seq data and MI GWAS data to reveal the mechanisms by which differential cell types influence myocardial infarction (MI) processing. Briefly, through the functional analysis and overlapping genes, integrating GWAS and single RNA-seq data, the function of pericyte may differ between cardiomyopathy and healthy individuals associated with MI (the workflow is shown in Figure 1).

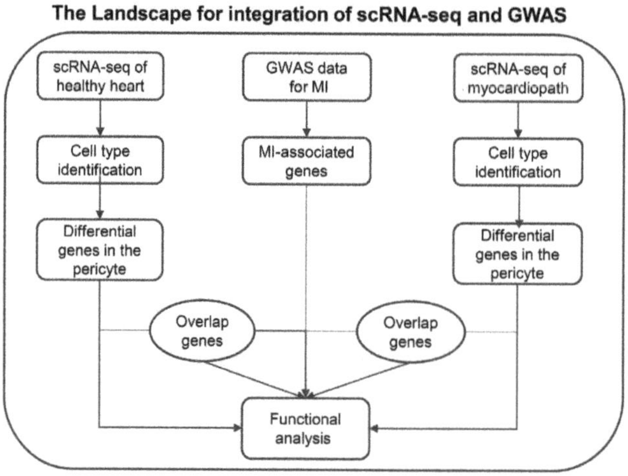

Figure 1. Introduction of the datasets and framework of analysis in this study.

2. Materials and Methods

2.1. Dataset Download

In this study, gene counts of single cells in the absence of overt cardiac disease were downloaded from the Broad Institute's Single Cell Portal (SCP498, accessed on August 2020) [19]. GWAS data for MI (myocardial infarction) were obtained from the GWAS Catalog GCST011365 [20]; another dataset of single cells from cardiomyopathy patients was accessed through the Broad Institute's Single Cell Portal (https://singlecell.broadinstitute.org/single_cell) under project ID SCP1303 (accessed on February 2021) [21]. There were 16 hearts from normal patients, 15 hearts from hypertrophic cardiomyopathy (HCM) patients, and 11 hearts from dilated cardiomyopathy (DCM) patients included in the following analysis.

2.2. Single-Cell RNA-Seq Analysis

The common processes of filtering, differential gene screening, dimensionality reduction, and clustering were carried out using the single-cell RNA-Seq analysis R package, Seurat (v.2.3.0) [22], according to a previous study. We screened cells in both single-cell experiments for those with fewer than 200 genes per 1000 UMIs to weed out low-quality cells, and eliminated cells with more than 5800 UMIs to weed out doublets that were more likely to exist. We used the Bioconductor developed by Lun et al. and implemented it in the R packages Scran (v.1.6.2) [23] and Scater (v.1.0.3) [24]. Principal component analysis was used to dimensionally reduce the expression matrix. The FindCluster function in Seurat used a graph-based clustering approach to identify clusters. In order to find rare populations, we used modularity-based clustering, a sensitive technique that occasionally over-partitions larger clusters. We used the model-based analysis of Single-cell Transcriptomics test for all single-cell differential expression tests.

2.3. Fine-Mapping

The causal variants were identified in the GWAS data. $p < 5 \times 10^{-8}$ was used as a filter to obtain loci with genome-wide significance. We used statistical fine-mapping across thousands of trait-associated loci, using a single evidence score to resolve association signals and connect each variant to its proximal and distal target genes. The Odds Ratio was used to evaluate the effect size of the MI GWAS data.

2.4. Pathway Enrichment Analysis

gProfiler (http://www.biit.cs.ut.ee/gprofiler/, accessed on 2007) was used for the pathway enrichment analysis. The Benjamini–Hochberg FDR was used to determine the significance threshold and 0.05 was used as a threshold in gProfiler. Gene Ontology (http://www.geneontology.org/, accessed on 2000), molecular pathways of Reactome (http://www.reactome.org/, accessed on 2005), and KEGG (https://www.genome.jp/kegg/, accessed on 1995) were applied to perform bioinformatics analysis.

2.5. Statistics

The differentially expressed genes were analyzed using the R package "limma" and defined as $p < 0.05$ and $|\log(FC)| > 1$. All results are shown as mean SEM. For comparisons between the two groups, a two-tailed, unpaired Student's *t*-test was used. In the present study, no randomization was used. $p < 0.05$ was used to define significant differences. Prism (version 9, San Diego, CA, USA) and R (version 4.1.2, New Zealand) software were used for the statistical analysis.

3. Results

3.1. Identifying Unique Genes and Function Pathways of Pericytes in Healthy Donors

To understand the proportion of different cell types in the heart, we used the scRNA-seq dataset of healthy donors to identify cell types (SCP498) [19]. A total of 17 distinct cell clusters were identified after unsupervised Louvain clustering at a resolution of 1.0. As present in Figure 2A,B, we showed cell cluster distributions using individual-specific uniform manifold approximation and projection representations. Then, we further analyzed the differential genes between these cells for each cell type, as shown in Figure 2C. We found that *DLC1/GUCY1A2/EGFLAM* were the top three uniquely expressed genes in the pericytes (Figure 2D). Also, we found that pericytes were concentrated in the left atrium and left ventricle tissues across several individuals (Figure 2E). Interestingly, we found that pericytes were involved in renin secretion, vascular smooth muscle contraction, gap junction, purine metabolism, and diabetic cardiomyopathy, according to the functional analysis ($p < 0.05$, Figure 2F).

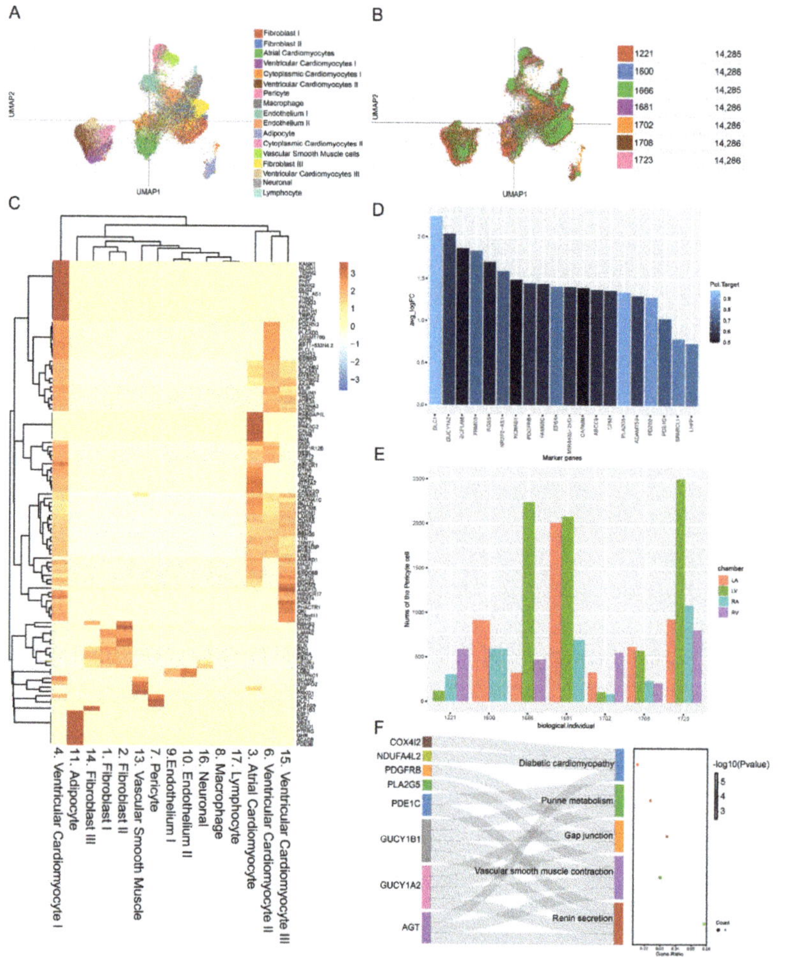

Figure 2. The single-cell landscape of healthy donors. (**A**) The cluster of the cell types in the hearts of healthy donors. (**B**) The cluster of the different individuals in the hearts of healthy donors. (**C**) The unique marker of the different cell types. (**D**) The average fold change of the marker gene in pericytes. (**E**) The number of pericytes across different chambers and individuals. (**F**) The functional enrichment for pericytes' marker genes. The greener the spot is, the more significant the statistical difference is ($p < 0.05$). LV, left ventricle; LA, left atrium; RA, right atrium; RV, right ventricle.

3.2. The Landscape of MI-Associated Genes

Although the mortality of MI is decreasing due to developments in medicine, MI still imposes a substantial disease burden on patients. How to improve the prevention and treatment of AMI remains a problem to be solved. The GWAS data of MI patients can help us understand the pathogenesis of MI. Through the GWAS data [20], we applied a fine-mapping technique to identify causal loci and then defined the nearest genes with each causal locus as MI-associated genes. Overall, we found 90 independent loci and 87 MI-associated genes ($p < 0.05$, Figure 3A,B). Then, we identified the pathways involved in these genes (Figure 3C). Among them, we found that the renin secretion and purine metabolism pathway were also found in the pathways of pericytes from healthy donors, which indicates the potential involvement of pericyte in the MI process. Furthermore, we found that MI-associated genes had a strong preference in the PPI (protein–protein interaction) network, according to the STRING database (Figure 3D). However, we did not find any overlap genes between the differential genes in healthy pericytes and MI-associated genes. This result reminds us that the dysfunction of pericytes may be involved in the MI process.

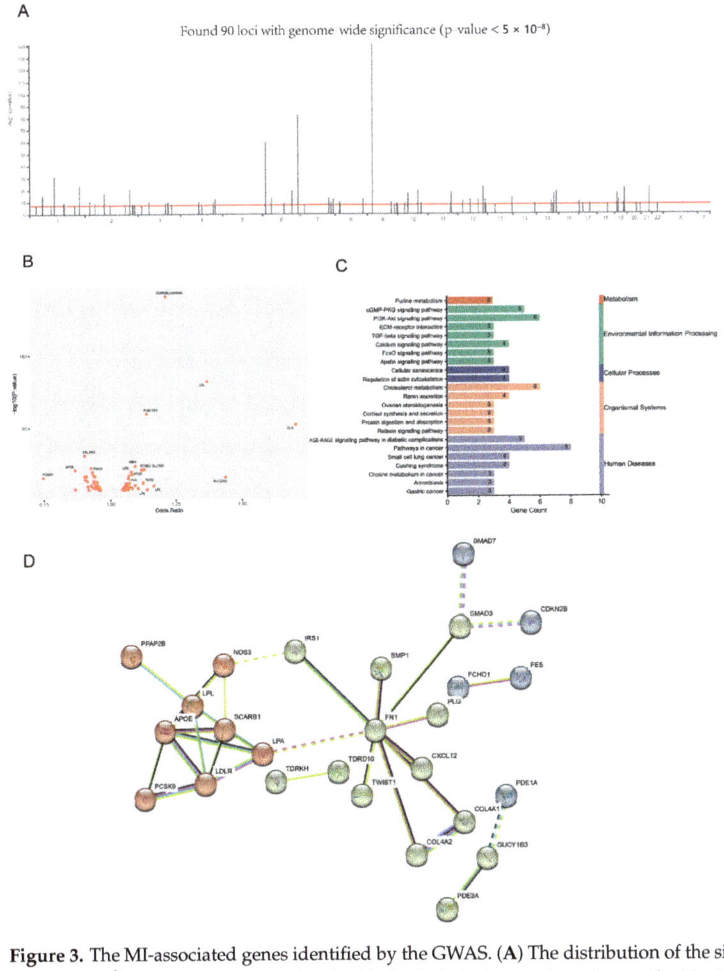

Figure 3. The MI-associated genes identified by the GWAS. (**A**) The distribution of the significant loci. ($p < 5 \times 10^{-8}$) (**B**) The genes associated with the loci; the larger the value on the Y-axis is, the more significant the statistical difference is. ($p < 0.05$). (**C**) The KEGG enrichment for the MI-associated genes. (**D**) The PPI network for the MI-associated genes.

3.3. *Identifying Function Pathways of Pericytes in Cardiomyopathy Patients*

Next, we tried to figure out the relationship between cardiomyopathy-associated MI and pericyte function. Thus, we used the single-cell RNA-seq of cardiomyopathy patients, a group associated with a potential cause of the poor long-term prognosis of MI [8,25], to identify the functional transformations in pericytes. Both HCM and DCM are the most common clinically observed cardiomyopathies. The physiopathology mechanisms of these two kinds of cardiomyopathies are not identical. Therefore, we analyzed the single-cell datasets from both HCM and DCM patients to reveal the function of pericytes in each (SCP1303) [21]. Firstly, we found 20 cell types across these datasets (Figure 4A). Then, comparing the percentages of different cell types among different disease groups, we found that Cardiomyocyte I, Fibroblast I, Endothelial I, Macrophage, and Pericyte I were the top five cell types in each disease group (Figure 4B). Cardiomyocyte I, Fibroblast I, Endothelial I, Macrophage, and Pericyte I were also the top six cell types in the number of significant genes (Figures 4C and 5A,B). According to the significant genes in each of these cell types, we conducted pathway enrichment analyses and compared them to those of normal patients. We found that signaling by interleukins, neutrophil degranulation, fatty acid metabolism, degradation of the extracellular matrix, and Y-Toxin signaling in the immune system were majorly negatively regulated in all cell types, and interestingly, biosynthesis of collagen, modulating enzymes, and collagen formation were uniquely negatively regulated in the pericytes ($p < 0.05$, Figure 5C). These results indicate that biosynthesis of collagen, modulating enzymes, and collagen formation may be the key pathways of pericytes in the pathophysiology of cardiac hypertrophy.

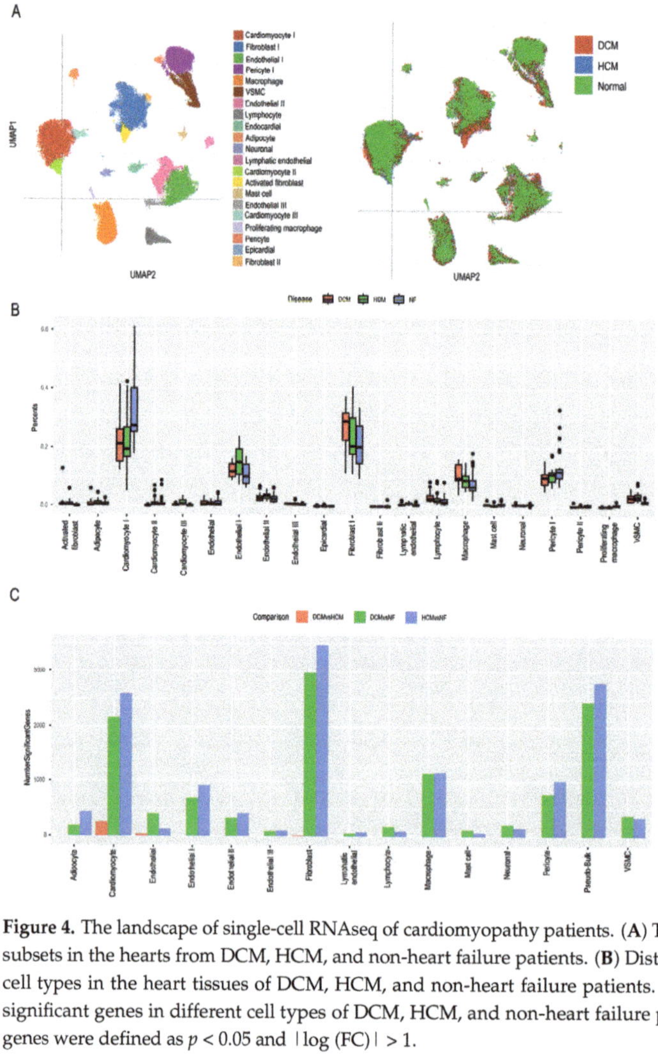

Figure 4. The landscape of single-cell RNAseq of cardiomyopathy patients. (**A**) The cluster of the cell subsets in the hearts from DCM, HCM, and non-heart failure patients. (**B**) Distribution of different cell types in the heart tissues of DCM, HCM, and non-heart failure patients. (**C**) The number of significant genes in different cell types of DCM, HCM, and non-heart failure patients. Significant genes were defined as $p < 0.05$ and $|\log(FC)| > 1$.

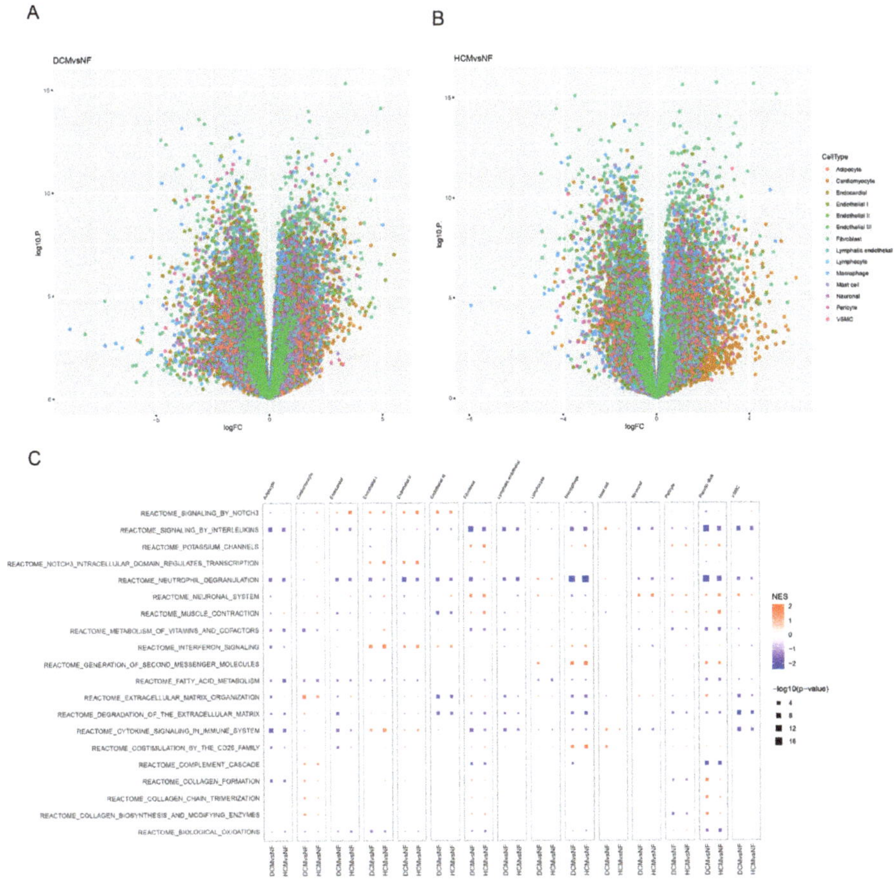

Figure 5. The function of the significant genes of cardiomyopathy patients in different cell types. (**A**) The volcano plot of the differential genes in different cell types between DCM and non-heart failure. Differential genes were defined as $p < 0.05$ and $|\log(\mathrm{FC})| > 1$. (**B**) The volcano plot of the differential genes in different cell types between HCM and non-heart failure. Differential genes were defined as $p < 0.05$ and $|\log(\mathrm{FC})| > 1$. (**C**) The gene enrichment for different cell types in different comparisons. The bigger the block, the more significant the statistical difference. ($p < 0.05$).

3.4. Hub Genes of Pericytes Involved in the MI Process

To further explore pericytes' function during the cardiomyopathy-associated MI process, we combined the MI GWAS dataset and single-cell RNA seq data from cardiomyopathy for analysis. We used differential genes to obtain cardiomyopathy-associated genes that overlapped with MI-associated genes (Figure 6A) in the top five cell types. We found that this overlap in genes was observed in Cardiomyocyte, Fibroblast, Pericyte, Macrophage, Lymphocyte, and Endocardial, varying from 1 to 13. Among them, the number of overlapping genes between the pericytes of cardiomyopathy and MI-associated genes was eight (Figure 6A). According to the functional analysis, enzyme-linked receptor protein signaling pathways, tube morphogenesis, pathways in cancer, epithelial to mesenchymal transition in colorectal cancer, and AGE−RAGE signaling pathways in diabetic complications were identified by these eight genes ($p < 0.05$, Figure 6B). PPI analysis found that the *COL4A2/COL4A1/SMAD3* genes were the hub genes of the pericytes involved in the MI process (Figure 6C). We found that the *COL4A2/COL4A1/SMAD3* were all expressed at lower levels in HCM and DCM patients but higher in pericytes (Figure 6D). These results may indicate that the regulation of the *COL4A2/COL4A1/SMAD3* pathway in pericytes may be a potential target that will affect the process of cardiomyopathy-associated MI.

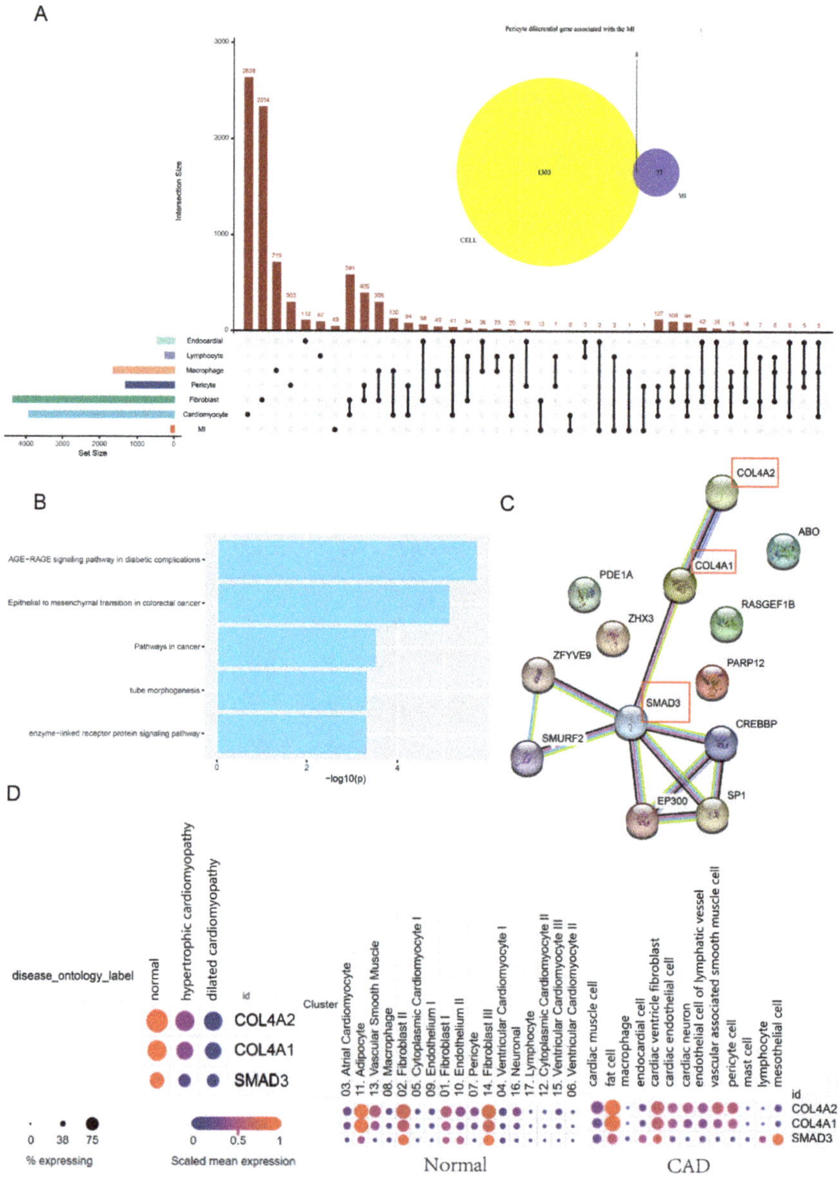

Figure 6. The integration of MI-associated genes and cardiomyopathy-associated genes. (**A**) The landscape of differential genes in different cell types overlapped with the MI-associated genes. (**B**) The gene enrichment for overlapping genes between pericytes and MI-associated genes. The larger the value on the X-axis, the more significant the statistical difference. ($p < 0.05$) (**C**) The hub genes for overlapping genes between pericytes and MI-associated genes. The red box showed the hub genes involved in the MI process. (**D**) The expression profile of hub genes across different disease statuses.

4. Discussion

Since their establishment in 2009, single-cell technologies have grown in popularity as their scale and cost have decreased significantly [26]. Single-cell techniques can be employed to answer a variety of questions, from determining the relationship between cell types and CVD to determining how gene expressions and regulations change in disease [27–30]. Several studies have used single-cell techniques to investigate AMI pathogenesis [29,31]. Jun Qian et al. discovered 27 cell clusters in 82,550 AMI patients' peripheral blood cells, including monocytes and T/B/NK cells [29]. Jun Qian et al. reported that *CCL5*, *TLR7*, and *CX3CR1* were significantly higher in patients with plaque rupture [29]. In addition, Song et al. defined a total of seven cell clusters marked by marker genes into five cell types and identified five hub genes involved in AMI progression (*ATM*, *CARM1*, *CASP8*, *CASP3*, and *PPARG*) using the scRNA-seq method [32]. In this study, we integrated single-cell RNA-seq data with MI GWAS data to reveal the mechanisms through which differentiated cell types influence cardiomyopathy-associated MI processing. We used scRNA-seq datasets from healthy donors to identify different cell types and their proportions in healthy hearts. In our research, a total of 17 distinct cell clusters were observed at a resolution of 1.0 after unsupervised Louvain clustering.

Microvascular pericytes are the cells that surround endothelial cells in capillaries and microvessels in most organs. The function of cardiac microvessels is important in keeping heart function and improving post-MI recovery. Cardiac-derived pericytes may be more prone to involvement in the function of cardiac microvessels. The gene heterogeneity among pericytes is very complicated, and in recent years, studies about pericyte function have been increasing. Single-cell analysis has revealed that pericytes make up a large proportion of the heart [13], implying that they play a vital role in the heart. It has been reported that cardiac pericytes can promote vascular homeostasis and attenuate adverse cardiac remodeling after AMI [17,18]. Additionally, the critical role of pericytes in the regulation of blood flow is widely recognized [33]. Augustin et al. found that the lack of pericyte-expressed Tie2 might lead to pro-migratory phenotype [34]. Moreover, it has been reported that the Ca^{2+} concentration of pericytes regulates TMEM16A and reduces post-ischemia blood flow [35]. However, studies on the relationship between pericytes and heart function are still limited until now.

A recent study from Teichmann et al. showed that pericytes account for a large proportion of the heart [13]. In this study, we found that pericytes from several individuals were mainly present in the left atrium and left ventricle tissues. In addition, *DLC1*/*GUCY1A2*/*EGFLAM* were found to be the top three uniquely expressed genes in pericytes. Zhang et al. utilized bioinformatics analysis to screen for biomarkers related to MI and revealed that *DLC1* is the most important node in MI [36]. So far, there is still a lack of study on the role of *DLC1* in pericytes. *EGFLAM* is found in a variety of organs and tissues, including the brain, endocrine tissue, and muscle tissue [37]. *EGFLAM* has been linked to defects in photoreceptor synapse function in congenital muscular dystrophies, such as muscle–eye–brain disorders caused by dystrophic glycosylation [38]. It has also been reported that *EGFLAM* can be a risk factor for dissecting aortic aneurysms [38]. An exome-wide association study identified *EGFLAM*, *SPATC1L*, and *RNASE13* as novel susceptibility loci for aortic aneurysms in the Japanese population [38]. In our research, we also found that pericytes in normal hearts are involved in renin secretion, vascular smooth muscle contraction, gap junctions, purine metabolism, and diabetic cardiomyopathy, according to functional analyses. It has been reported that ACE2 is highly expressed in heart pericytes, inducing microvascular dysfunction [39]. This study suggests that the renin–angiotensin system and related genes are important to pericyte function. We found that renin secretion and purine metabolism are also present in the MI pathway through the GWAS, suggesting that pericytes have the potential to participate in the MI process.

Cardiomyopathy complicated by MI is relevant to a poor prognosis. Both cardiomyopathy and MI can evolve into heart failure. To study the pathogenesis of cardiomyopathy-associated MI in depth, we compared the percentages of different cell types in the different disease groups (HCM and DCM) in the database [21]. Cardiomyocyte I, Fibroblast I, Endothelial I, Macrophage, and Pericyte I were the top five cell types in each disease group. Signaling by interleukins, neutrophil degranulation, fatty acid metabolism, degradation of the extracellular Matrix, and Y-toxin signaling in the immune system were uniquely negatively regulated in all cell types. The extracellular matrix consists of collagen, elastin, fibronectin, and other proteoglycans, which are vital for damage repair and signal transduction. It was reported that collagen plays a special role in maintaining the integrity of blood vessels and in the processes of thrombosis and scarring [40]. Collagen fibers, in addition to providing tensile strength and stiffness to the heart muscle, also serve as structural scaffolding for muscle cells. According to several studies, coronary occlusion not only kills muscle cells but also destroys collagen [40]. Thus, collagen damage impairs muscle cell support, reduces myocardial strength and stiffness, and allows infarcted tissue to expand. The extracellular matrix metalloproteinases degrade collagen, which is normally dormant in the myocardium but is activated by ischemia [41]. The number of damaged collagen fibers in the rat heart increased over time after coronary occlusion, within the first four days after infarction, as measured by light microscopy [42]. All these results indicate that collagen may be meaningful to cardiomyopathy-complicated MI. Next, we used differential genes from cardiomyopathy patients to obtain genes that overlapped with MI-associated genes in the top five cell types. Eight genes were identified and several pathways were discovered through functional analysis. It seems that the EMT could improve the prognosis of MI patients. According to recent research, EMT is involved in the process of cardiac regeneration and repair [43,44]. Hence, changes in EMT-related genes might explain the poor prognosis of cardiomyopathy-associated MI.

Our further PPI analysis found that the *COL4A2/COL4A1/SMAD3* genes are the central genes of pericytes involved in the MI process. We found that the expression of *COL4A2/COL4A1/SMAD3* was lower in both HCM and DCM, but higher in pericytes, which may suggest that pericytes can prevent the progression of MI by upregulating *COL4A2/COL4A1/SMAD3*. *COL4A1* and *COL4A2* encode the first and second chains of type IV collagen [45,46]. Type IV collagen is a critical component of basement membrane integrity and functionality [47]. Mutations in the *COL4A1/COL4A2* locus influence vascular cell survival, atherosclerotic plaque stability, and MI risk [48]. Apoptosis is induced by the silencing of *COL4A1* or *COL4A2* in vascular smooth muscle cells or endothelial cells. Similarly, shift mutations in *COL4A2* increase the rate of apoptosis in fibroblasts of mutation-carrying individuals [48]. So far, no study has proposed the effect of *COL4A1* or *COL4A2* on cardiomyopathy-associated MI. Smad2 and Smad3 signaling pathways located in cardiomyocytes and stromal cells are activated in infarcted myocardium [49]. Smad3 signal transduction enhances myofibroblast transdifferentiation and stimulates matrix preservation procedures [50]. In reperfusion infarct models, there is a total absence of Smad3 attenuating post-infarct remolding. The negative effects of Smad3 deletion include uncontrolled fibroblast proliferation and a misaligned myofibroblast array in the marginal region [51]. Smad3 signaling controls fibroblast activity and triggers integrin-mediated NOX2 expression. The infarcted heart is shielded from the effects of post-infarct dysfunction by the absence of cardiomyocyte-specific Smad3 [51,52]. Smad3 loss is related to reduced NOX2 levels, nitrosation stress, and MMP2 expression, which promotes the survival and growth of B cells, as well as the weakening of cardiomyocyte apoptosis in remodeled myocardium [51]. Additionally, Smad3-expressing macrophages guard the infarcted heart, promote phagocytosis, and control inflammation [53]. Additionally, Smad3 is crucial in the process of cardiomyopathy initiation and development. The expression of Smad2 and Smad3 aggravates myocardial fibrosis, and the abnormal regulation of the Smad pathway leads to more cardiac deaths [54]. Disturbing EphrinB2, which inhibits the TGF-β/Smad3 pathway in fibroblasts, can reduce fibrotic remodeling and improve heart function in cardiomyopathy models [55]. All these studies suggest that the *COL4A2/COL4A1/SMAD3* pathway may have a potential function in regulating the progress of cardiomyopathy-associated MI. However, how the *COL4A2/COL4A1/SMAD3* pathway regulates the process of cardiomyopathy-associated MI requires further study.

5. Conclusions

Overall, in this study, we integrated single-cell data from normal and CVD individual, along with MI GWAS data to reveal the function of pericytes in the cardiomyopathy-associated MI process. Using single-cell data from healthy donors, we found that pericytes were concentrated in the left atrium and left ventricle tissues across several individuals. Interestingly, we found that pericytes were involved in renin secretion, vascular smooth muscle contraction, gap junction, purine metabolism, and diabetic cardiomyopathy, according to the functional analysis. Next, MI-associated genes were identified through the GWAS data. Moreover, we found that the pericytes were the top five cell types in each disease group. Finally, we identified *COL4A2/COL4A1/SMAD3* as the hub gene in pericyte function involved in the cardiomyopathy-associated MI process. We believe this study provides new evidence proving that pericytes play a key role in the pathogenesis of cardiomyopathy-associated MI and could serve as potential therapy targets for the treatment of patients with cardiomyopathy-associated MI.

6. Limitations

However, the limitations of this study should not be overlooked. Firstly, this research was a secondary analysis of published single-cell sequencing databases and a GWAS database, which may cause certain deviations in the results. Secondly, the single-cell sequencing data of cardiomyopathy were not matched with the GWAS data of MI. It would be better to analyze data from patients with cardiomyopathy-associated MI directly, rather than combining two different datasets. Finally, the bioinformatics analysis only provided potential pathways involved in cardiomyopathy-associated MI. These results still need further verification through additional experiments.

Author Contributions: B.H. and L.S. provided the conception and supervised the progress. Y.L. and H.H. contributed to the design of the study and the first draft. F.L. contributed to the data analysis. J.X., Y.M. and L.F. contributed to revising the manuscript. All authors have read and agreed to the published version of the manuscript.

Funding: The project was supported by grants from the National Natural Science Foundation of China (numbers 81830010, 82130012), Clinical Research Plan of SHDC (number SHDC2020CR1039B), Emerging and Advanced Technology Programs of Hospital Development Center of Shanghai (number: SHDC12018129).

Institutional Review Board Statement: Not applicable.

Informed Consent Statement: Not applicable.

Data Availability Statement: The datasets analyzed during the current study are available in the Broad Institute's Single Cell Portal (SCP498, SCP1303) and GWAS Catalog GCST011365. All the original data are available from the corresponding author.

Acknowledgments: We are grateful to everyone who contributed to this study.

Conflicts of Interest: The authors declare that this study was conducted in the absence of any commercial or financial relationships that could be construed as a potential conflict of interest.

Abbreviations

CVD	cardiovascular disease
AMI	acute myocardial infarction
MI	myocardial infarction
PPI	protein–protein interaction
HCM	hypertrophic cardiomyopathy

DCM	dilated cardiomyopathy
EMT	epithelial–mesenchymal transition
LV	left ventricle
LA	left atrium
RA	right atrium
RV	right ventricle

References

1. Roth, G.A.; Mensah, G.A.; Johnson, C.O.; Addolorato, G.; Ammirati, E.; Baddour, L.M.; Barengo, N.C.; Beaton, A.Z.; Benjamin, E.J.; Benziger, C.P.; et al. Global Burden of Cardiovascular Diseases and Risk Factors, 1990–2019: Update from the GBD 2019 Study. *J. Am. Coll. Cardiol.* **2020**, *76*, 2982–3021. [CrossRef] [PubMed]
2. Hung, M.J.; Cheng, C.W.; Yang, N.I.; Hung, M.Y.; Cherng, W.J. Coronary vasospasm-induced acute coronary syndrome complicated by life-threatening cardiac arrhythmias in patients without hemodynamically significant coronary artery disease. *Int. J. Cardiol.* **2007**, *117*, 37–44. [CrossRef] [PubMed]
3. Tibaut, M.; Mekis, D.; Petrovic, D. Pathophysiology of Myocardial Infarction and Acute Management Strategies. *Cardiovasc. Hematol. Agents Med. Chem.* **2017**, *14*, 150–159. [CrossRef] [PubMed]
4. Westman, P.C.; Lipinski, M.J.; Luger, D.; Waksman, R.; Bonow, R.O.; Wu, E.; Epstein, S.E. Inflammation as a Driver of Adverse Left Ventricular Remodeling after Acute Myocardial Infarction. *J. Am. Coll. Cardiol.* **2016**, *67*, 2050–2060. [CrossRef] [PubMed]
5. Abdallah, M.H.; Arnaout, S.; Karrowni, W.; Dakik, H.A. The management of acute myocardial infarction in developing countries. *Int. J. Cardiol.* **2006**, *111*, 189–194. [CrossRef]
6. Shi, X.; Zhang, X.; Zhuang, F.; Lu, Y.; Liang, F.; Zhao, N.; Wang, X.; Li, Y.; Cai, Z.; Wu, Z.; et al. Congestive heart failure detection based on attention mechanism-enabled bi-directional long short-term memory model in the internet of medical things. *J. Ind. Inf. Integr.* **2022**, *30*, 100402. [CrossRef]
7. Reddy, K.; Khaliq, A.; Henning, R.J. Recent advances in the diagnosis and treatment of acute myocardial infarction. *World J. Cardiol.* **2015**, *7*, 243–276. [CrossRef]
8. Liu, F.; Ma, Y.; Ge, H.; Zhao, Y.; Shen, H.; Zhang, D.; Sun, Y.; Ma, X.; Cheng, Y.; Zhou, Y. Long-Term Outcomes of Acute Myocardial Infarction in Patients with Hypertrophic Cardiomyopathy. *Angiology* **2018**, *69*, 900–908. [CrossRef]
9. Jia, D.; Chen, S.; Bai, P.; Luo, C.; Liu, J.; Sun, A.; Ge, J. Cardiac Resident Macrophage-Derived Legumain Improves Cardiac Repair by Promoting Clearance and Degradation of Apoptotic Cardiomyocytes After Myocardial Infarction. *Circulation* **2022**, *145*, 1542–1556. [CrossRef]
10. Shi, X.; Cao, Y.; Zhang, X.; Gu, C.; Liang, F.; Xue, J.; Ni, H.W.; Wang, Z.; Li, Y.; Wang, X.; et al. Comprehensive Analysis of N6-Methyladenosine RNA Methylation Regulators Expression Identify Distinct Molecular Subtypes of Myocardial Infarction. *Front. Cell Dev. Biol.* **2021**, *9*, 756483. [CrossRef]
11. Zhao, M.; Nakada, Y.; Wei, Y.; Bian, W.; Chu, Y.; Borovjagin, A.V.; Xie, M.; Zhu, W.; Nguyen, T.; Zhou, Y.; et al. Cyclin D2 Overexpression Enhances the Efficacy of Human Induced Pluripotent Stem Cell-Derived Cardiomyocytes for Myocardial Repair in a Swine Model of Myocardial Infarction. *Circulation* **2021**, *144*, 210–228. [CrossRef] [PubMed]
12. Craig, D.J.; James, A.W.; Wang, Y.; Tavian, M.; Crisan, M.; Péault, B.M. Blood Vessel Resident Human Stem Cells in Health and Disease. *Stem Cells Transl. Med.* **2022**, *11*, 35–43. [CrossRef] [PubMed]
13. Litviňuková, M.; Talavera-López, C.; Maatz, H.; Reichart, D.; Worth, C.L.; Lindberg, E.L.; Kanda, M.; Polanski, K.; Heinig, M.; Lee, M.; et al. Cells of the adult human heart. *Nature* **2020**, *588*, 466–472. [CrossRef] [PubMed]
14. Su, H.; Cantrell, A.C.; Zeng, H.; Zhu, S.H.; Chen, J.X. Emerging Role of Pericytes and Their Secretome in the Heart. *Cells* **2021**, *10*, 548. [CrossRef] [PubMed]
15. Spencer, H.L.; Jover, E.; Cathery, W.; Avolio, E.; Rodriguez-Arabaolaza, I.; Thomas, A.C.; Alvino, V.V.; Sala-Newby, G.; Dang, Z.; Fagnano, M.; et al. Role of TPBG (Trophoblast Glycoprotein) Antigen in Human Pericyte Migratory and Angiogenic Activity. *Arterioscler. Thromb. Vasc. Biol.* **2019**, *39*, 1113–1124. [CrossRef]
16. Yoshida, Y.; Kabara, M.; Kano, K.; Horiuchi, K.; Hayasaka, T.; Tomita, Y.; Takehara, N.; Minoshima, A.; Aonuma, T.; Maruyama, K.; et al. Capillary-resident EphA7(+) pericytes are multipotent cells with anti-ischemic effects through capillary formation. *Stem Cells Transl. Med.* **2020**, *9*, 120–130. [CrossRef]
17. Quijada, P.; Park, S.; Zhao, P.; Kolluri, K.S.; Wong, D.; Shih, K.D.; Fang, K.; Pezhouman, A.; Wang, L.; Daraei, A.; et al. Cardiac pericytes mediate the remodeling response to myocardial infarction. *J. Clin. Investig.* **2023**, *133*, e162188. [CrossRef]
18. Alex, L.; Tuleta, I.; Hernandez, S.C.; Hanna, A.; Venugopal, H.; Astorkia, M.; Humeres, C.; Kubota, A.; Su, K.; Zheng, D.; et al. Cardiac Pericytes Acquire a Fibrogenic Phenotype and Contribute to Vascular Maturation After Myocardial Infarction. *Circulation* **2023**, *148*, 882–898. [CrossRef]
19. Tucker, N.R.; Chaffin, M.; Fleming, S.J.; Hall, A.W.; Parsons, V.A.; Bedi, K.C., Jr.; Akkad, A.D.; Herndon, C.N.; Arduini, A.; Papangeli, I.; et al. Transcriptional and Cellular Diversity of the Human Heart. *Circulation* **2020**, *142*, 466–482. [CrossRef]
20. Hartiala, J.A.; Han, Y.; Jia, Q.; Hilser, J.R.; Huang, P.; Gukasyan, J.; Schwartzman, W.S.; Cai, Z.; Biswas, S.; Trégouët, D.A.; et al. Genome-wide analysis identifies novel susceptibility loci for myocardial infarction. *Eur. Heart J.* **2021**, *42*, 919–933. [CrossRef]

21. Chaffin, M.; Papangeli, I.; Simonson, B.; Akkad, A.D.; Hill, M.C.; Arduini, A.; Fleming, S.J.; Melanson, M.; Hayat, S.; Kost-Alimova, M.; et al. Single-nucleus profiling of human dilated and hypertrophic cardiomyopathy. *Nature* **2022**, *608*, 174–180. [CrossRef] [PubMed]
22. Ramachandran, P.; Dobie, R.; Wilson-Kanamori, J.R.; Dora, E.F.; Henderson, B.E.P.; Luu, N.T.; Portman, J.R.; Matchett, K.P.; Brice, M.; Marwick, J.A.; et al. Resolving the fibrotic niche of human liver cirrhosis at single-cell level. *Nature* **2019**, *575*, 512–518. [CrossRef] [PubMed]
23. Lun, A.T.; McCarthy, D.J.; Marioni, J.C. A step-by-step workflow for low-level analysis of single-cell RNA-seq data with Bioconductor. *F1000Research* **2016**, *5*, 2122. [CrossRef]
24. McCarthy, D.J.; Campbell, K.R.; Lun, A.T.; Wills, Q.F. Scater: Pre-processing, quality control, normalization and visualization of single-cell RNA-seq data in R. *Bioinformatics* **2017**, *33*, 1179–1186. [CrossRef] [PubMed]
25. Yang, Y.J.; Fan, C.M.; Yuan, J.Q.; Zhang, H.B.; Duan, F.J.; Wang, Z.M.; Guo, X.Y.; Zhai, S.S.; An, S.Y.; Hang, F.; et al. Long-term survival after acute myocardial infarction in patients with hypertrophic cardiomyopathy. *Clin. Cardiol.* **2017**, *40*, 26–31. [CrossRef]
26. Hwang, B.; Lee, J.H.; Bang, D. Single-cell RNA sequencing technologies and bioinformatics pipelines. *Exp. Mol. Med.* **2018**, *50*, 96. [CrossRef]
27. Iqbal, F.; Lupieri, A.; Aikawa, M.; Aikawa, E. Harnessing Single-Cell RNA Sequencing to Better Understand How Diseased Cells Behave the Way They Do in Cardiovascular Disease. *Arterioscler. Thromb. Vasc. Biol.* **2021**, *41*, 585–600. [CrossRef]
28. Paik, D.T.; Cho, S.; Tian, L.; Chang, H.Y.; Wu, J.C. Single-cell RNA sequencing in cardiovascular development, disease and medicine. *Nat. Rev. Cardiol.* **2020**, *17*, 457–473. [CrossRef]
29. Qian, J.; Gao, Y.; Lai, Y.; Ye, Z.; Yao, Y.; Ding, K.; Tong, J.; Lin, H.; Zhu, G.; Yu, Y.; et al. Single-Cell RNA Sequencing of Peripheral Blood Mononuclear Cells from Acute Myocardial Infarction. *Front. Immunol.* **2022**, *13*, 908815. [CrossRef]
30. Shi, X.; Zhang, L.; Li, Y.; Xue, J.; Liang, F.; Ni, H.W.; Wang, X.; Cai, Z.; Shen, L.H.; Huang, T.; et al. Integrative Analysis of Bulk and Single-Cell RNA Sequencing Data Reveals Cell Types Involved in Heart Failure. *Front. Bioeng. Biotechnol.* **2021**, *9*, 779225. [CrossRef]
31. Jin, K.; Gao, S.; Yang, P.; Guo, R.; Li, D.; Zhang, Y.; Lu, X.; Fan, G.; Fan, X. Single-Cell RNA Sequencing Reveals the Temporal Diversity and Dynamics of Cardiac Immunity after Myocardial Infarction. *Small Methods* **2022**, *6*, e2100752. [CrossRef] [PubMed]
32. Song, Z.; Gao, P.; Zhong, X.; Li, M.; Wang, M.; Song, X. Identification of Five Hub Genes Based on Single-Cell RNA Sequencing Data and Network Pharmacology in Patients with Acute Myocardial Infarction. *Front. Public Health* **2022**, *10*, 894129. [CrossRef]
33. Longden, T.A.; Zhao, G.; Hariharan, A.; Lederer, W.J. Pericytes and the Control of Blood Flow in Brain and Heart. *Annu. Rev. Physiol.* **2023**, *85*, 137–164. [CrossRef] [PubMed]
34. Teichert, M.; Milde, L.; Holm, A.; Stanicek, L.; Gengenbacher, N.; Savant, S.; Ruckdeschel, T.; Hasanov, Z.; Srivastava, K.; Hu, J.; et al. Pericyte-expressed Tie2 controls angiogenesis and vessel maturation. *Nat. Commun.* **2017**, *8*, 16106. [CrossRef] [PubMed]
35. Korte, N.; Ilkan, Z.; Pearson, C.L.; Pfeiffer, T.; Singhal, P.; Rock, J.R.; Sethi, H.; Gill, D.; Attwell, D.; Tammaro, P. The Ca^{2+}-gated channel TMEM16A amplifies capillary pericyte contraction and reduces cerebral blood flow after ischemia. *J. Clin. Investig.* **2022**, *132*, e154118. [CrossRef]
36. Zhang, G.; Li, J.; Sun, H.; Yang, G. Screening for the Biomarkers Associated with Myocardial Infarction by Bioinformatics Analysis. *J. Comput. Biol.* **2020**, *27*, 779–785. [CrossRef]
37. Chen, J.; Zhang, J.; Hong, L.; Zhou, Y. EGFLAM correlates with cell proliferation, migration, invasion and poor prognosis in glioblastoma. *Cancer Biomark.* **2019**, *24*, 343–350. [CrossRef]
38. Yamada, Y.; Sakuma, J.; Takeuchi, I.; Yasukochi, Y.; Kato, K.; Oguri, M.; Fujimaki, T.; Horibe, H.; Muramatsu, M.; Sawabe, M.; et al. Identification of EGFLAM, SPATC1L and RNASE13 as novel susceptibility loci for aortic aneurysm in Japanese individuals by exome-wide association studies. *Int. J. Mol. Med.* **2017**, *39*, 1091–1100. [CrossRef]
39. Chen, L.; Li, X.; Chen, M.; Feng, Y.; Xiong, C. The ACE2 expression in human heart indicates new potential mechanism of heart injury among patients infected with SARS-CoV-2. *Cardiovasc. Res.* **2020**, *116*, 1097–1100. [CrossRef]
40. Peuhkurinen, K.; Risteli, L.; Jounela, A.; Risteli, J. Changes in interstitial collagen metabolism during acute myocardial infarction treated with streptokinase or tissue plasminogen activator. *Am. Heart J.* **1996**, *131*, 7–13. [CrossRef]
41. Frangogiannis, N.G. The extracellular matrix in myocardial injury, repair, and remodeling. *J. Clin. Investig.* **2017**, *127*, 1600–1612. [CrossRef] [PubMed]
42. Basso, C.; Thiene, G.; Della Barbera, M.; Angelini, A.; Kirchengast, M.; Iliceto, S. Endothelin A-receptor antagonist administration immediately after experimental myocardial infarction with reperfusion does not affect scar healing in dogs. *Cardiovasc. Res.* **2002**, *55*, 113–121. [CrossRef] [PubMed]
43. Aharonov, A.; Shakked, A.; Umansky, K.B.; Savidor, A.; Genzelinakh, A.; Kain, D.; Lendengolts, D.; Revach, O.Y.; Morikawa, Y.; Dong, J.; et al. ERBB2 drives YAP activation and EMT-like processes during cardiac regeneration. *Nat. Cell Biol.* **2020**, *22*, 1346–1356. [CrossRef] [PubMed]
44. Blom, J.N.; Feng, Q. Cardiac repair by epicardial EMT: Current targets and a potential role for the primary cilium. *Pharmacol. Ther.* **2018**, *186*, 114–129. [CrossRef]
45. Poschl, E.; Pollner, R.; Kuhn, K. The genes for the alpha 1(IV) and alpha 2(IV) chains of human basement membrane collagen type IV are arranged head-to-head and separated by a bidirectional promoter of unique structure. *EMBO J.* **1988**, *7*, 2687–2695. [CrossRef]

46. Yang, W.; Ng, F.L.; Chan, K.; Pu, X.; Poston, R.N.; Ren, M.; An, W.; Zhang, R.; Wu, J.; Yan, S.; et al. Coronary-Heart-Disease-Associated Genetic Variant at the COL4A1/COL4A2 Locus Affects COL4A1/COL4A2 Expression, Vascular Cell Survival, Atherosclerotic Plaque Stability and Risk of Myocardial Infarction. *PLoS Genet.* **2016**, *12*, e1006127. [CrossRef]
47. Yurchenco, P.D. Basement membranes: Cell scaffoldings and signaling platforms. *Cold Spring Harb. Perspect. Biol.* **2011**, *3*, a004911. [CrossRef]
48. Verbeek, E.; Meuwissen, M.E.; Verheijen, F.W.; Govaert, P.P.; Licht, D.J.; Kuo, D.S.; Poulton, C.J.; Schot, R.; Lequin, M.H.; Dudink, J.; et al. COL4A2 mutation associated with familial porencephaly and small-vessel disease. *Eur. J. Hum. Genet.* **2012**, *20*, 844–851. [CrossRef]
49. Hao, J.; Ju, H.; Zhao, S.; Junaid, A.; Scammell-La Fleur, T.; Dixon, I.M. Elevation of expression of Smads 2, 3, and 4, decorin and TGF-beta in the chronic phase of myocardial infarct scar healing. *J. Mol. Cell. Cardiol.* **1999**, *31*, 667–678. [CrossRef]
50. Dobaczewski, M.; Bujak, M.; Li, N.; Gonzalez-Quesada, C.; Mendoza, L.H.; Wang, X.F.; Frangogiannis, N.G. Smad3 signaling critically regulates fibroblast phenotype and function in healing myocardial infarction. *Circ. Res.* **2010**, *107*, 418–428. [CrossRef]
51. Kong, P.; Shinde, A.V.; Su, Y.; Russo, I.; Chen, B.; Saxena, A.; Conway, S.J.; Graff, J.M.; Frangogiannis, N.G. Opposing Actions of Fibroblast and Cardiomyocyte Smad3 Signaling in the Infarcted Myocardium. *Circulation* **2018**, *137*, 707–724. [CrossRef] [PubMed]
52. Bujak, M.; Ren, G.; Kweon, H.J.; Dobaczewski, M.; Reddy, A.; Taffet, G.; Wang, X.F.; Frangogiannis, N.G. Essential role of Smad3 in infarct healing and in the pathogenesis of cardiac remodeling. *Circulation* **2007**, *116*, 2127–2138. [CrossRef] [PubMed]
53. Chen, B.; Huang, S.; Su, Y.; Wu, Y.J.; Hanna, A.; Brickshawana, A.; Graff, J.; Frangogiannis, N.G. Macrophage Smad3 Protects the Infarcted Heart, Stimulating Phagocytosis and Regulating Inflammation. *Circ. Res.* **2019**, *125*, 55–70. [CrossRef] [PubMed]
54. Zhang, Z.; Zhang, F.; Zhang, M.; Xue, H.; Fan, L.; Weng, Y. The role of SMAD signaling in hypertrophic obstructive cardiomyopathy: An immunohistopathological study in pediatric and adult patients. *Sci. Rep.* **2023**, *13*, 3706. [CrossRef]
55. Su, S.A.; Yang, D.; Wu, Y.; Xie, Y.; Zhu, W.; Cai, Z.; Shen, J.; Fu, Z.; Wang, Y.; Jia, L.; et al. EphrinB2 Regulates Cardiac Fibrosis Through Modulating the Interaction of Stat3 and TGF-β/Smad3 Signaling. *Circ. Res.* **2017**, *121*, 617–627. [CrossRef]

biomedicines

MDPI

Opinion

The Negative Impact of Insulin Resistance/Hyperinsulinemia on Chronic Heart Failure and the Potential Benefits of Its Screening and Treatment

Serafino Fazio [1,*], Valentina Mercurio [2], Flora Affuso [3] and Paolo Bellavite [4,*]

1 Department of Internal Medicine, University of Naples Federico II, 80138 Naples, Italy
2 Department of Translational Medical Sciences, University of Naples Federico II, 80131 Naples, Italy; valemercurio@yahoo.com
3 Independent Researcher, 73014 Lecce, Italy; floraaffuso@libero.it
4 Homeopathic Medical School of Verona, 37121 Verona, Italy
* Correspondence: fazio0502@gmail.com (S.F.); paolo.bellavite@gmail.com (P.B.)

Abstract: This opinion article highlights the potential alterations caused by insulin resistance and hyperinsulinemia on the cardiovascular system and their negative impact on heart failure (HF), and describes the potential benefits of an early screening with consequent prompt treatment. HF is the final event of several different cardiovascular diseases. Its incidence has been increasing over the last decades because of increased survival from ischemic heart disease thanks to improvements in its treatment (including myocardial revascularization interventions) and the increase in life span. In particular, incidence of HF with preserved ejection fraction (HFpEF) is significantly increasing, and patients with HFpEF often are also affected by diabetes mellitus and insulin resistance (IR), with a prevalence > 45%. Concentric left ventricular (LV) remodeling and diastolic dysfunction are the main structural abnormalities that characterize HFpEF. It is well documented in the literature that IR with chronic hyperinsulinemia, besides causing type 2 diabetes mellitus, can cause numerous cardiovascular alterations, including endothelial dysfunction and increased wall thicknesses of the left ventricle with concentric remodeling and diastolic dysfunction. Therefore, it is conceivable that IR might play a major role in the pathophysiology and the progressive worsening of HF. To date, several substances have been shown to reduce IR/hyperinsulinemia and have beneficial clinical effects in patients with HF, including SGLT2 inhibitors, metformin, and berberine. For this reason, an early screening of IR could be advisable in subjects at risk and in patients with heart failure, to promptly intervene with appropriate therapy. Future studies aimed at comparing the efficacy of the substances used both alone and in association are needed.

Keywords: diabetes; heart failure; insulin resistance; hyperinsulinemia; SGLT2 inhibitors; metformin; berberine

1. Introduction

Chronic heart failure (HF) represents the final clinical evolution common to several cardiovascular diseases characterized by different specific etiology and pathophysiology. HF is the leading cause of hospitalizations in individuals aged >65 years. The crude age-adjusted incidence ranges from 1 to 5 cases per thousand person-years, and there is an exponential increase in incidence with advancing age. Its prevalence ranges from 3 to 20 individuals per 1000 people over 65 years of age.

Chronic HF is still burdened by high mortality: only 35% of patients are alive 5 years after the first diagnosis of HF. The mortality of subjects with HF is 6–7 times higher than the general population in the same age group [1]. Insulin resistance (IR)/hyperinsulinemia (Hyperins) is a pathogenic factor of type 2 diabetes, associated with metabolic syndrome, hypertension, low HDL cholesterol, and hypertriglyceridemia, but may also be present in a significant proportion of healthy subjects of normal weight. It affects about 40% of the population in Western countries and is associated with incident symptomatic cardiovascular disease [2].

Chronic HF has been classified into three different phenotypes based on the values of the measured left ventricular ejection fraction (LVEF):

I. Heart failure with reduced ejection fraction (HFrEF) is defined by an LVEF $\leq$ 40%.
II. Heart failure with mildly reduced EF (HFmrEF) is defined by an EF between 41% and 49%.
III. Heart failure with preserved EF (HFpEF) is defined by an LVEF $\geq$ 50% in the presence of symptoms and signs of HF associated with structural and/or functional cardiac abnormalities and/or increased natriuretic peptides [1].

HFpEF accounts for about 45% of all HF cases and has been on the rise in the recent years [3]. In fact, due to the increased scientific interest in HF and improved characterization and modern diagnostic tools, the incidence of HFrEF tends to decrease in percentage, while HFpEF tends to increase [4].

Increased left ventricular mass (LVM) is a stronger predictor of HF than coronary artery calcium score [5]. Increased LVM, as measured by echocardiogram, was also found to be an independent risk factor of a depressed EF [6]. The majority of patients with HFpEF show a concentric pattern of LV remodeling, characterized mainly by: A. Normal or near normal LV end-diastolic volume; B. Increased parietal thickness and/or LVM; C. Increased ratio of LVM to cavity volume; D. Increased relative wall thickness (RWT) defined as 2$\times$ posterior wall thickness (PWT)/LV end-diastolic diameter (LVDD), or as septal WT+PWT/LVDD [3]. The most common cause of HFpEF is diastolic LV dysfunction, secondary to increased stiffness of a hypertrophied LV causing elevation of LV filling pressures.

Data from clinical studies show that diabetes mellitus (DM) has a prevalence of about 45% in individuals with HFpEF, but IR certainly has a higher prevalence [7]. Generalized IR is strictly associated with HF, and this increases the risk of hospitalization, cardiovascular deaths, and all-cause deaths. The changes in insulin signaling, due to IR, within cardiomyocytes and vascular smooth muscle cells alter cardiac function, thereby worsening HF [8].

In this opinion article, we describe the potential alterations caused by IR/Hyperins on the cardiovascular system, highlighting its negative impact in HF, and discuss the possibility of early screening and treatment of IR to improve prognosis in HF patients. In this regard, we reviewed the scientific literature, selecting articles on PubMed, Scopus, and Science Direct using the following key terms: heart failure, cardiovascular system, insulin resistance, hyperinsulinemia, diabetes mellitus, treatment of insulin resistance, SGLT2 Inhibitors, metformin, berberine, GLP-1 receptor agonists. We collected and analyzed laboratory and clinical research studies describing the effects of IR/Hyperins on the cardiovascular system, and more specifically in HF. Furthermore, we analyzed the manuscripts describing the potential beneficial effects of reducing IR/Hyperins through treatment with some known substances.

2. Insulin Resistance/Hyperinsulinemia and Chronic Heart Failure

IR is a pathological condition characterized by a decrease in sensitivity and response to the metabolic actions of insulin. In fact, at a given concentration of this hormone, the biological effects are clearly less than expected. Increased insulin levels (hyperinsulinemia) are necessary in order to maintain normal glucose tolerance and, therefore, hyperinsulinemia is a defining event of IR [9,10].

IR turns out to be a key mechanism in the development of type 2 diabetes, systemic hypertension, HF, and other various cardiovascular diseases. IR is the earliest abnormality in the natural history of type 2 diabetes, due to defects of insulin receptor function, and the chronic insulin over-secretion results in progressive pancreatic beta cell dysfunction [9,10]. Some studies have shown that hyperinsulinemia, resulting from IR, anticipates the development of overt type 2 diabetes by as much as 10 to 15 years. In the majority of cases, IR is asymptomatic or paucisymptomatic, and affected subjects, when identified, are mostly referred for lifestyle modifications with frequent non-adherence to such indications [9,10]. While it can be easily suspected in the context of metabolic syndrome and polycystic ovary syndrome, the diagnosis of IR/Hyperins becomes difficult in the case of normal-weight or thin subjects. The diagnosis, however, should be done as early as possible to initiate prompt therapeutic interventions.

The diagnostic gold standard for IR is the hyperinsulinemic euglycemic clamp, but this test is poorly applicable for screening purposes, because of its difficulty, time of performance and cost. For clinical screening, several easier-to-obtain substitute indices have been evaluated, such as the Homeostasis Model Assessment of IR index (HOMA-IR) and the Triglyceride–Glucose Index (TyG). HOMA-IR is calculated by multiplying the fasting blood glucose value in mmol/L $\times$ the fasting insulinemia value in mU/L and dividing the result by 22.5 [(glycemia $\times$ insulinemia)/22.5]. The TyG index is obtained by calculating the natural logarithm of the product between the fasting triglyceride (Tg) value in mg/dl and the fasting blood sugar (FBG) value in mg/dl, then dividing the result by 2 [logn (serum Tg $\times$ FBG)/2]. Both indices showed good correlation with clamp data. A HOMA-IR index between 0.23 and 2.5 can be considered normal in the adult population, while the cut-off value for the TyG index is 4.5 [11,12].

Chronic long-lasting hyperinsulinemia, typical of IR, produces damage in target organs, and one of the recognized targets of insulin is certainly the cardiovascular system [13]. Indeed, insulin exerts various pathophysiological actions on the heart and vessels, since insulin receptors are highly expressed in the myocardiocytes and vascular smooth muscle cells. Insulin signaling regulates heart growth, survival, substrate uptake and utilization, and mitochondrial metabolism. Consequently, impaired insulin signaling may contribute to the development of pathological ventricular remodeling and progression of HF [14].

Insulin is also a growth factor, and both insulin and insulin like growth factor-1 (IGF-1) are able to bind to and activate each other's receptors, even if with lower affinity. Both the insulin receptor (InsR) and the IGF-1 receptor (IGF-1 R) elicit a common downstream signaling resulting in the activation, by phosphorylation of a tyrosine kinase, of two important pathways: that of phosphoinositide-3 kinase (PI3K/Akt), and that of Shc-Ras-mitogen activated protein kinase (MAPK) [15]. The PI3K/Akt pathway is an intracellular signal transduction pathway that promotes important actions in response to extracellular signals, but predominantly mediates the metabolic actions of insulin, regulating glucose metabolism in muscle and in adipose and hepatic tissues; it also regulates nitric oxide (NO) formation by vascular endothelial and smooth muscle cells. The MAPKs are among the most ancient signal transduction pathways which coordinately regulate gene expression, mitosis, survival, apoptosis, differentiation, etc. and primarily mediate mitogenic and proliferative actions of insulin; furthermore, they stimulate endothelial cells to form increased amounts of the vasoconstrictor endothelin-1(ET-1) and increase the expression of adhesion molecules on the vascular endothelium [16,17]. Under normal conditions, these two pathways are in balance and help to maintain vascular homeostasis: the first pathway, stimulating NO production, causes vasodilatation and reduction in vascular resistance with increased blood flow to tissues, while the second one, stimulating ET-1 formation, causes vasoconstriction and activates the sympathetic system, leading to a hypertensive pattern and accelerating the development of cardiac hypertrophy and atherosclerosis.

The main mechanisms by which IR/Hyperins lead to left ventricular failure are summarized in Figure 1.

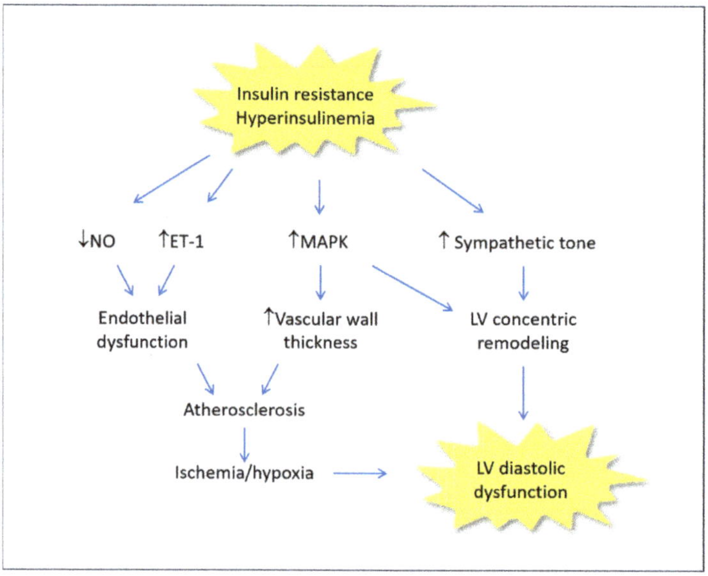

Figure 1. Molecular mechanisms involved in the cardiac consequences of insulin resistance and hyperinsulinemia. ET-1: Endothelin-1; LV: Left ventricle; MAPK: Mitogen-activated protein kinase; NO: Nitric oxide.

Under conditions of IR, the PI3K-dependent pathway is specifically altered while the MAPK-dependent pathway is altered little or not at all. This is why the hyperinsulinemia that is typically associated with IR, in an attempt to maintain glucose levels in the normal range, ends up increasing the activity of the MAPK pathway, with prevalence of deleterious effects at the cardiovascular level due to mitogenic and proliferative actions, and to over exposure to ET-1, which, in the presence of reduced NO production, results in serious endothelial dysfunction [18]. Chronic hyperinsulinemia can result in arterial hypertension not only for the elevated levels of ET-1 and the increased sympathetic tone, but also for a documented anti natriuretic effect of insulin [19]. In addition, chronically increased insulin levels may produce mitogenic and proliferative effects on the cardiovascular system, as they result in proliferation of vascular smooth muscle cells and increased LVM with concentric remodeling [20]. As mentioned above, the cardiovascular changes produced by hyperinsulinemia may act misrecognized for years in the presence of IR until overt type 2 diabetes appears. For this reason, most individuals who develop overt type 2 diabetes after years of IR, already show evident cardiovascular abnormalities at first diagnosis, such that, according to guidelines, they are subject to a higher degree of severity in cardiovascular prevention and treatment lines [21].

Alzadjali et al. (2009) [22] demonstrated how IR is highly prevalent among non-diabetic HF patients (67%). In such patients, the fasting IR index increased progressively with worsening New York Heart Association classes. In addition, patients with HF and IR demonstrated significantly reduced exercise capacity and peak O_2 achieved, compared with patients with HF alone. Unfortunately, no distinction was made between patients with HFrEF and patients with HFpEF in this study [22]. There is a large scientific literature highlighting that IR/Hyperins is associated with pathological remodeling of the LV. It is well known that LVH is a constant feature of diabetic cardiomyopathy [23]. In fact, LVH is very prevalent in patients with type 2 diabetes and is a strong predictor of cardiovascular adverse events, in particular of HFpEF. LVH can result in impediment to normal LV filling and can lead to diastolic HF [24]. In these cases, intervention with drugs such as angiotensin-converting enzyme inhibitors, sartans, etc., which result in LVH reduction, also improves the prognosis of this condition [25]. However, the causes of LVH in subjects with diabetes are not fully elucidated. Some researchers have hypothesized and demonstrated that increased fat deposition in the LV myocardium may also contribute to the increased ventricular mass, and that excess lipid in the myocardiocytes may alter cell signaling and cardiac structure by accumulation of toxic lipid species (lipotoxicity), resulting in abnormal heart function [26–28]. Other researchers have shown that IR/Hyperins and waist-to-hip ratio are associated with LV concentric remodeling regardless of BMI levels, suggesting that treating IR could give a greater boost to the regression of LV concentric remodeling and improve the prognosis regarding the development of HF [29]. Diabetes is associated with an increased risk of morbidity and mortality in patients with HFrEF, HFmrEF, and, especially, in patients with HFpEF. DM in patients with HFpEF is associated with a 2-fold increase in the risk of cardiovascular death and HF-related hospitalizations, and with an increased risk of all-cause mortality [30,31]. In the digoxin study, DM was found to be associated with a 68% increased risk of HF hospitalization and death [32]. This was later confirmed in the I-Preserve study [33]. In the RELAX study, it was shown that subjects with HFpEF and DM had similar levels of NT-ProBNP compared with nondiabetics, but markedly higher levels of the vasoconstrictor endothelin-1 (ET-1), of markers of inflammation such as uric acid and C-reactive protein, and of profibrotic markers such as valectin-3 and carboxy-terminal telopeptide of collagen type 1 [34]. It is well known that the alterations of these parameters are also characteristic of IR/Hyperin states [35]. Echocardiographically, patients with HF and DM had a significantly abnormal LV diastolic function as shown by higher E/e′ ratio, with increased LVM and reduced exercise tolerance compared with subjects with HF without DM [36].

Recently, it has been reported that, due to the advancement in HF treatment, a relevant number of patients with HFrEF and HFmrEF have experienced an improvement of LVEF, such that it is almost back to normal value. This condition has been termed HF with recovered EF (HFrecEF). We have seen how IR is highly present in the subjects with HF and is closely related to prognosis. Patients with HF and IR had significantly greater difficulty in improving their LVEF, and so the authors conclude that IR is independently associated with a failure to improve LVEF in subjects with HFrEF [37]. It is well known that patients with type 2 DM have longstanding IR/Hyperins before they reach the stage of overt DM, and this contributes to much of the pathologic cardiovascular changes already present in the diabetic subjects at first diagnosis.

3. Treatment of Insulin Resistance/Hyperinsulinemia: Possible Beneficial Effects in Patients with Chronic HF

The metabolic and organic imbalances described are very complex and there are many different therapeutic approaches that may be considered for the treatment of IR/Hyperins.

3.1. Role of Diet

The gold standard for the treatment of IR/Hyperins is certainly constituted by following a balanced diet, low in carbohydrates, low in calories in obese and overweight subjects, and physical activity, when possible, moderate and constant [38]. Among the various diets, very low-calorie ketogenic diets (VLCKDs), which have been used with good results in obese or overweight subjects with prediabetes or diabetes, deserve special mention. VLCKDs are calorie-restricted diets (<800 Kcal/day but >600 Kcal/day) with a low carbohydrate content (between 20 and 60 g/day). According to international guidelines, VLCKDs can be used continuously for 12 weeks, always under medical supervision [39].

When the intake of carbohydrates is drastically reduced, the consequent modification of the relationship between the concentration of insulin and that of glucagon promotes the mobilization of lipids from tissue deposits and the oxidation for energy purposes.

In practice, the drastic reduction in the intake of carbohydrates determines an increase in fat catabolism, with an imbalance between the production of pyruvate, oxaloacetate and acetyl-Coenzyme A (acetyl-CoA). Excess acetyl-CoA is transformed in the liver cells into the three ketone bodies: acetoacetate, hydroxybutyrate, and acetone. Myocardium, skeletal muscle, and brain capture and can use the first two. At the pancreatic level, these contribute to metabolic improvement in patients with IR.

Normally, the heart's large demand for energy is met mainly by the mitochondrial oxidation of fatty acids and glucose. In HF, there is a reduction in mitochondrial oxidative metabolism and glucose oxidation, which makes the heart starved of energy. Ketone bodies can be rapidly oxidized by the heart muscle and can provide a replacement and additional energy source to the failing heart. This mechanism may become an adaptive response of the heart to reduce the severity of HF [40].

However, as is well known from clinical practice, maintaining a correct lifestyle is consistently performed only by a low percentage of patients, while the majority, after a variable duration, return to a detrimental lifestyle. To improve adherence to these indications, patients must be well informed, and reminded often, of the risks they incur by not adhering to these indications. Furthermore, we are also convinced that, to reduce hospital admissions of patients for HF exacerbation, they must be followed consistently at home via telemedicine or through a periodic monthly visit by a nurse specialized in caring for patients with HF [41].

3.2. Sodium-Glucose Cotransporter-2 Inhibitors

Sodium-glucose cotransporter-2 (SGLT2) inhibitors are a class of oral drugs approved by the US FDA for use with diet and exercise to lower blood sugar in adult patients with type2 diabetes and recently included in the guidelines for treatment of HF [1]. They include canaglifozin, dapaglifozin, and empaglifozin. It has been shown that treatment with SGLT2 inhibitors reduces the risk of hospitalization, death from cardiovascular events, and all-cause mortality in patients with HF [42]. In a recent study, 6263 patients > 40 years of age with an EF > 40%, assigned to receive dapaglifozin (10 mg once a day) or placebo in addition to standard therapy, showed a significant reduction in the combined risk of worsening HF and death from cardiovascular events. This result was similar in both patients with EF $\geq$ 60% and those with EF < 60% [43]. This beneficial effect of SGLT2 inhibitors in patients with HFpEF has also been confirmed by a recent meta-analysis study performed on 12,251 patients drawn from the DELIVER and EMPEROR-Preserved studies. Indeed, it shows that treatment with SGLT2 inhibitors results in a consistent reduction in both deaths from cardiovascular events and first hospitalization for HF [44]. The exact mechanisms by which these drugs beneficially act in HF remain elusive. However, the suggested mechanisms are: blood volume regulation, cardiorenal mechanisms, metabolic effects, improved cardiac remodeling, direct effects on contractility and sodium ion homeostasis, reduction of inflammation and oxidative stress, etc. [45]. Administration of an SGLT2 inhibitor to subjects with IR/Hyperins reduces the amount of glucose disposal required to maintain blood glucose in the normal range as result of increased urinary glucose excretion. Therefore, the amount of insulin required for a given amount of glucose disposal will be reduced. As a consequence, average circulating insulin levels will be lower than before treatment [46]. SGLT2 inhibitors reduce IR and circulating insulin levels, thereby reducing their adverse cardiovascular effects. Cardiac remodeling is a constant component of IR/Hyperins and an important determinant of the development and progression of HF. Counteracting pathological cardiac remodeling is likely to be a central mechanism in determining the cardioprotective benefits of SGLT2 inhibitors.

Treatment with SGLT2 inhibitors has been shown to favorably affect cardiac remodeling through myocardial, mitochondrial, interstitial, vascular, autonomic nervous system, etc. applications [47]. Results of a meta-analysis study of randomized and controlled trials, comparing the effects of SGLT2 inhibitor treatment versus placebo on changes in LVM, assessed by cardiac magnetic resonance imaging, showed that such therapy significantly reduced LVM [48]. In particular, the reduction in LVM and concentric remodeling produce an improvement of diastolic function and an increase in EF. Very recently, some researchers have reported that a treatment of six months with dapaglifozin in 27 patients with type 2

DM significantly reduced the epicardial adipose tissue thickness (evaluated by echocardiography), HbA$_1$c, body weight, BMI, and blood glucose, while the LV global longitudinal strain (evaluated as an index of LV systolic function by m-mode echocardiography) was increased. These data further support the beneficial effects of SGLT2 inhibitors on the heart, although all of these effects have to be confirmed in the long term [49]. In addition, 12 large-scale trials involving more than 70,000 patients with HF showed that long-term SGLT2 inhibition produced a relevant 20 to 25% decrease in the combined risk of cardiovascular deaths or hospitalizations for HF, providing insights unto the durability and sustainability of their effects [50]. Due to their beneficial effects on the outcomes of patients with HF, SGLT2 inhibitors have entered the guidelines for the treatment of HF. However, further studies are needed to monitor any long-term adverse effects.

3.3. *Metformin*

Metformin, an oral antidiabetic belonging to the biguanide class and used for many years in the treatment of type 2 diabetes mellitus, has been amply demonstrated to reduce IR/Hyperins and has shown beneficial effects in patients with HFpEF. In fact, the results of a review and meta-regression analysis study have shown that treatment with metformin reduces mortality in patients with HF, although larger positive effects ($p < 0.003$) were demonstrated in the subgroup of patients with HFpEF [51]. Indeed, metformin has been shown to have numerous favorable effects in HF patients, such as, for example, the improvement of myocardial energy status consequent to modulation of glucose and lipid metabolism, the reduction in oxidative stress and inflammation, and the reduction in cardiac pathologic remodeling [52]. Oxidative stress and inflammation are mechanisms and significant drivers in the development and progression of cardiovascular diseases. Experimental and clinical studies have demonstrated that oxidative stress and inflammation associated with conditions of IR, such as obesity, hypertension, and diabetes produce LV hypertrophy, fibrosis, diastolic dysfunction, HF, and ischemia/reperfusion damage [53]. Therefore, it seems obvious that determining a reduction in these parameters can produce a series of beneficial effects at the cardiovascular level. A recent meta-analysis has shown that metformin treatment results in favorable effects on LVM and LVEF, both in patients with and those without pre-existing cardiovascular disease [54]. Few years ago, another interesting study, double-blind and placebo-controlled, showed that, in non-diabetic but insulin resistant patients with HF, metformin treatment for 4 months produced a significant ($p < 0.001$) improvement in IR indices, accompanied by a significant ($p < 0.036$) reduction in the minute ventilation/carbon dioxide production (VE/VCO_2) slope [55]. The VE/VCO_2 slope has a strong predictive value in patients with HF, and the risk of mortality is thought to increase significantly when the value is >32.8 [56].

3.4. *Berberine*

Many natural substances have shown beneficial effects on IR/Hyperins. Some studies demonstrated the beneficial effects of berberine, quercetin, and silymarin on IR/Hyperins and the cardiovascular system. From the analysis of experimental in vitro and in vivo studies, it clearly appears that these three substances reduce IR and consequent circulating elevated insulin levels. Therefore, these substances could protect the evolution toward overt type 2 diabetes and the development of cardiovascular abnormalities [35]. Both quercetin and silymarin have extensive literature that support their efficacy in counteracting IR/Hyperins and LVH development, and in preventing cardiovascular alterations [57–65]. However, these experimental studies have not been followed by clinical studies to confirm their beneficial effects in humans. Berberine, in contrast, has many clinical studies supporting its efficacy in counteracting IR/Hyperins and, consequently, in protecting against the development of IR-related cardiovascular damage.

Berberine is a vegetable alkaloid in use for over 2000 years in Chinese and Ayurvedic medicines, which has been shown to have numerous beneficial effects on human health. It is contained in numerous plants, including *Hydrastis canadensis* and *Coptis chinensis*. A study designed to assess the efficacy of berberine to produce improvements in patients with HF, was carried out on patients with HF divided into two groups: a group of 79 patients treated with berberine and a group of 76 patients treated with a placebo in addition to standard therapy, according to guidelines, for HF. Evaluation of the parameters considered was done basally, after 8 weeks and after an average of 24 months of follow-up. Berberine treatment produced a significant increase in EF and exercise capacity and a reduction in the frequency and complexity of ventricular premature beats. In addition, during the 2-year follow-up, 7 patients died in the berberine group and 13 patients in the placebo group ($p < 0.02$) [66].

A further study evaluated the relationship between the clinical effects of berberine at a dose of 1.2 g per day in patients with severe congestive HF and the hematic concentrations of berberine assessed by HPLC. It was shown that berberine decreased the number and complexity of premature ventricular beats and increased EF more in patients whose plasma concentration of berberine was >0.11 mg/L than in those with lower concentrations [67]. In a randomized, double-blind, placebo-controlled trial of 18 weeks, 59 patients with metabolic syndrome were treated with a nutraceutical combination containing 500 mg of berberine or with placebo once daily. The results showed a significant decrease ($p < 0.05$) in HOMA-IR and fasting insulin levels in the berberine-treated group [68]. Also, these patients showed a significant decrease in LVM, RWT, and diastolic dysfunction, evaluated by Doppler-echocardiography, after treatment in comparison with the placebo group [68]. These results were confirmed by a further multicenter, randomized, double-blind, placebo-controlled trial performed in 145 patients with metabolic syndrome and LVH. The patients were divided into two groups; the first group of 74 patients was given a nutraceutical combination containing berberine at 500 mg daily, and the second group (71 patients) were given a placebo. The duration of the trial was six months. The results showed that the treated group had a significant reduction in LVM ($p < 0.001$) as compared with the placebo group. The authors concluded that the treatment could represent an effective strategy to reduce the cardiovascular risk [69]. Unfortunately, despite the beneficial effects demonstrated at the cardiovascular level by these substances both in experimental studies and in some clinical studies, they have so far not been taken into consideration for a trial demonstrating clear clinical efficacy in patients with HF.

3.5. Glucagon-like Peptide-1 Receptor Agonists

Glucagon-like peptide-1 is a hormone produced by the intestine that stimulates insulin secretion and inhibits glucagon secretion by the pancreas. Among other things, it slows down gastric emptying, increasing the sense of satiety, and reduces appetite by acting directly on the hunger regulation centers in the central nervous system, thus helping to lose weight [70].

Glucagon-like peptide-1 receptor agonists (GLP-1 RAs) are substances utilized in the treatment of type 2 diabetes and obesity. The ones currently in use are: semaglutide, albiglutide, delaglutide, exenatide, liraglutide and lixisenatide. Despite the positive reports on the beneficial effects of treatment with GLP-1 RAs in the treatment of diabetes and obesity, the data in the scientific literature on the use of GLP-1 RAs in subjects with HF are contrasting. In fact, a recent meta-analysis study of 54,092 participants of 7 randomized controlled trials on the use of GLP-1 RAs in subjects with type 2 diabetes, of whom 16% also had a history of HF, showed that these drugs may help prevent new onset of HF in the diabetic population, while, on the other hand, in subjects with pre-existing HF, they did not reduce the risk of HF exacerbation or mortality [71]. A further recent meta-analysis study, performed to verify whether the use of GLP-1 RAs in patients with HF with or without type 2 diabetes could improve morbidity and mortality compared to placebo treatment, also demonstrated that the GLP-1 RAs did not lead to an improvement in major adverse cardiovascular events, including cardiovascular mortality, or a reduction in hospitalizations for HF. Furthermore, they did not determine an improvement in EF and in the six-minute walking test [72].

3.6. Interactions of Some Drugs, Used in HF, with IR/Hyperins

Some older drugs, still quite often used by patients with HF, while improving the overall prognosis of these patients, can induce or worsen a state of IR/Hyperins. The drugs most commonly used are beta-blockers, thiazide diuretics, and statins. The beta-blockers that have a greater negative action on IR/Hyperins are predominantly those of the first generation, not beta 1 selective and without vasodilating action, such as propranolol [73,74]. As far as thiazide diuretics are concerned, the negative action on IR/Hyperins has been abundantly confirmed, particularly at high doses, which are most commonly used in HF states [75–77]. Statins are drugs widely used in cardiovascular prevention for the treatment of hypercholesterolemia. Their efficacy on cardiovascular morbidity and mortality has been sufficiently demonstrated, and this justifies their use. However, they can determine or worsen a state of IR/Hyperins, which, as we have seen, can have a negative effect on the cardiovascular system and partially reduce the positive action of statins [78]. Probably, their cardiovascular prevention action would be even more positive if they did not have this negative action towards IR. What has been said should lead us to contrast the potential negative action of these drugs against IR/Hyperins, where possible, with lifestyle changes and with the use of substances that have demonstrated efficacy against IR/Hyperins. This could determine a favorable synergistic action that could add efficacy to their positive action on cardiovascular morbidity and mortality.

4. Conclusions

Despite the considerable progress in the prevention and treatment of heart diseases, HF is still a very important cause of recurring hospitalizations, with relevant social and health care costs, and it is burdened with a significant mortality. It is also noteworthy, not only for treatment purposes, to highlight the increase in the incidence of heart failure. Among the causes that could have contributed to this increase could be the increase in the incidence of IR and consequent hyperinsulinemia, and diabetes. It is known that IR is closely related to metabolic syndrome, which is in a phase of progressive diffusion and increase in developed and developing countries. Elevated circulating insulin levels from IR could contribute to the development and progressive worsening of HF. In fact, a considerable prevalence of IR has been demonstrated in HF. Hyperinsulinemia, as amply demonstrated in the scientific literature, can, over the years, cause progressive alterations at the cardiovascular level. For this reason, early screening of IR/Hyperins in at-risk subjects and in patients with HF could certainly be useful, given that we now have numerous substances that have been shown to be able to counteract it and, probably, reduce and slow down the progression toward type 2 diabetes and cardiovascular damage. What the best drug and the correct dosage might be, or whether it is better to use a combination of drugs, is not currently known. For these reasons, dose-response trials and head-to-head comparisons are necessary to help optimize the treatment.

Author Contributions: Conceptualization, S.F., F.A. and P.B.; methodology, V.M.; writing—original draft preparation, S.F., F.A.; writing—review and editing, V.M. and P.B. All authors have read and agreed to the published version of the manuscript.

Funding: This research received no external funding.

Institutional Review Board Statement: Not applicable.

Informed Consent Statement: Not applicable.

Data Availability Statement: Data sharing not applicable.

Conflicts of Interest: P.B. has a consultation with Vanda Omeopatici s.r.l. (Roma, Frascati), a company which produces food supplements, but that company had no role in the design of the study; in the collection, analyses, or interpretation of data; in the writing of the manuscript; or in the decision to publish the results. The other authors have no potential conflicts of interest to declare.

References

1. McDonagh, T.A.; Metra, M.; Adamo, M.; Gardner, R.S.; Baumbach, A.; Böhm, M.; Burri, H.; Butler, J.; Čelutkienė, J.; Chioncel, O.; et al. 2023 Focused Update of the 2021 ESC Guidelines for the diagnosis and treatment of acute and chronic heart failure. *Eur. Heart J.* **2023**, *44*, 3627–3639. [CrossRef]
2. Bonora, E.; Kiechl, S.; Willeit, J.; Oberhollenzer, F.; Egger, G.; Meigs, J.B.; Bonadonna, R.C.; Muggeo, M. Insulin resistance as estimated by homeostasis model assessment predicts incident symptomatic cardiovascular disease in caucasian subjects from the general population: The Bruneck study. *Diabetes Care* **2007**, *30*, 318–324. [CrossRef] [PubMed]
3. Ma, C.; Luo, H.; Fan, L.; Liu, X.; Gao, C. Heart failure with preserved ejection fraction: An update on pathophysiology, diagnosis, treatment, and prognosis. *Braz. J. Med. Biol. Res.* **2020**, *53*, e9646. [CrossRef]
4. Naing, P.; Forrester, D.; Kangaharan, N.; Muthumala, A.; Myint, S.M.; Playford, D. Heart failure with preserved ejection fraction: A growing global epidemic. *Aust. J. Gen. Pract.* **2019**, *48*, 465–471. [CrossRef]
5. Kawel-Boehm, N.; Kronmal, R.; Eng, J.; Folsom, A.; Burke, G.; Carr, J.J.; Shea, S.; Lima, J.A.C.; Bluemke, D.A.; O'brien, C.; et al. Left Ventricular Mass at MRI and Long-term Risk of Cardiovascular Events: The Multi-Ethnic Study of Atherosclerosis (MESA). *Radiology* **2019**, *293*, 107–114. [CrossRef] [PubMed]
6. Drazner, M.H.; Rame, J.; Marino, E.K.; Gottdiener, J.S.; Kitzman, D.W.; Gardin, J.M.; Manolio, T.A.; Dries, D.L.; Siscovick, D.S. Increased left ventricular mass is a risk factor for the development of a depressed left ventricular ejection fraction within five years: The Cardiovascular Health Study. *J. Am. Coll. Cardiol.* **2004**, *43*, 2207–2215. [CrossRef] [PubMed]
7. McHugh, K.; DeVore, A.D.; Wu, J.; Matsouaka, R.A.; Fonarow, G.C.; Heidenreich, P.A.; Yancy, C.W.; Green, J.B.; Altman, N.; Hernandez, A.F. Heart Failure with Preserved Ejection Fraction and Diabetes: JACC State-of-the-Art Review. *J. Am. Coll. Cardiol.* **2019**, *73*, 602–611. [CrossRef]
8. Riehle, C.; Abel, E.D. Insulin Signaling and Heart Failure. *Circ. Res.* **2016**, *118*, 1151–1169. [CrossRef] [PubMed]
9. Freeman, A.M.; Pennings, N. Insulin Resistance. In *StatPearls*; StatPearls: Treasure Island, FL, USA, 2023.
10. Lebovitz, H.E. Insulin resistance: Definition and consequences. *Exp. Clin. Endocrinol. Diabetes* **2001**, *109* (Suppl. S2), S135–S148. [CrossRef] [PubMed]
11. Ziaee, A.; Esmailzadehha, N.; Oveisi, S.; Ghorbani, A.; Ghanei, L. The threshold value of homeostasis model assessment for insulin resistance in Qazvin Metabolic Diseases Study (QMDS): Assessment of metabolic syndrome. *J. Res. Health Sci.* **2015**, *15*, 94–100. [PubMed]
12. Guerrero-Romero, F.; Simental-Mendía, L.E.; González-Ortiz, M.; Martínez-Abundis, E.; Ramos-Zavala, M.G.; Hernández-González, S.O.; Jacques-Camarena, O.; Rodríguez-Morán, M. The Product of Triglycerides and Glucose, a Simple Measure of Insulin Sensitivity. Comparison with the Euglycemic-Hyperinsulinemic Clamp. *J. Clin. Endocrinol. Metab.* **2010**, *95*, 3347–3351. [CrossRef] [PubMed]
13. Ginsberg, H.N. Insulin resistance and cardiovascular disease. *J. Clin. Investig.* **2000**, *106*, 453–458. [CrossRef] [PubMed]
14. Abel, E.D. Insulin signaling in the heart. *Am. J. Physiol. Endocrinol. Metab.* **2021**, *321*, E130–E145. [CrossRef]
15. Cai, W.; Sakaguchi, M.; Kleinridders, A.; Pino, G.G.-D.; Dreyfuss, J.M.; O'neill, B.T.; Ramirez, A.K.; Pan, H.; Winnay, J.N.; Boucher, J.; et al. Domain-dependent effects of insulin and IGF-1 receptors on signalling and gene expression. *Nat. Commun.* **2017**, *8*, 14892. [CrossRef]
16. Chopra, I.; Li, H.F.; Wang, H.; Webster, K.A. Phosphorylation of the insulin receptor by AMP-activated protein kinase (AMPK) promotes ligand-independent activation of the insulin signalling pathway in rodent muscle. *Diabetologia* **2012**, *55*, 783–794. [CrossRef] [PubMed]
17. Petersen, M.C.; Shulman, G.I. Mechanisms of Insulin Action and Insulin Resistance. *Physiol. Rev.* **2018**, *98*, 2133–2223. [CrossRef]
18. Mercurio, V.; Carlomagno, G.; Fazio, V.; Fazio, S. Insulin resistance: Is it time for primary prevention? *World J. Cardiol.* **2012**, *4*, 1–7. [CrossRef]
19. Bachmann, K.N.; Deger, S.M.; Alsouqi, A.; Huang, S.; Xu, M.; Ferguson, J.F.; Su, Y.R.; Niswender, K.D.; Ikizler, T.A.; Wang, T.J. Acute effects of insulin on circulating natriuretic peptide levels in humans. *PLoS ONE* **2018**, *13*, e0196869. [CrossRef] [PubMed]
20. Stout, R.W. Insulin as a mitogenic factor: Role in the pathogenesis of cardiovascular disease. *Am. J. Med.* **1991**, *90*, S62–S65. [CrossRef]
21. Buse, J.B.; Ginsberg, H.N.; Bakris, G.L.; Clark, N.G.; Costa, F.; Fonseca, V.; Grundy, S.; Nesto, R.W.; Porte, D.; Eckel, R.; et al. Primary prevention of cardiovascular diseases in people with diabetes mellitus: A scientific statement from the American Heart Association and the American Diabetes Association. *Circulation* **2007**, *115*, 114–126. [CrossRef]
22. Alzadjali, M.A.; Godfrey, V.; Khan, F.; Choy, A.; Doney, A.S.; Wong, A.K.; Petrie, J.R.; Struthers, A.D.; Lang, C.C. Insulin Resistance Is Highly Prevalent and Is Associated with Reduced Exercise Tolerance in Nondiabetic Patients with Heart Failure. *J. Am. Coll. Cardiol.* **2009**, *53*, 747–753. [CrossRef]
23. Mohan, M.; Dihoum, A.; Mordi, I.R.; Choy, A.-M.; Rena, G.; Lang, C.C. Left Ventricular Hypertrophy in Diabetic Cardiomyopathy: A Target for Intervention. *Front. Cardiovasc. Med.* **2021**, *8*, 746382. [CrossRef] [PubMed]
24. Palmieri, V.; Russo, C.; Bella, J.N. Treatment of isolated left ventricular diastolic dysfunction in hypertension: Reaching blood pressure target matters. *Hypertension* **2010**, *55*, 224–225. [CrossRef] [PubMed]
25. Tai, C.; Gan, T.; Zou, L.; Sun, Y.; Zhang, Y.; Chen, W.; Li, J.; Zhang, J.; Xu, Y.; Lu, H.; et al. Effect of angiotensin-converting enzyme inhibitors and angiotensin II receptor blockers on cardiovascular events in patients with heart failure: A meta-analysis of randomized controlled trials. *BMC Cardiovasc. Disord.* **2017**, *17*, 257. [CrossRef]

26. Ormazabal, V.; Nair, S.; Elfeky, O.; Aguayo, C.; Salomon, C.; Zuñiga, F.A. Association between insulin resistance and the development of cardiovascular disease. *Cardiovasc. Diabetol.* **2018**, *17*, 122. [CrossRef] [PubMed]
27. Levelt, E.; Mahmod, M.; Piechnik, S.K.; Ariga, R.; Francis, J.M.; Rodgers, C.T.; Clarke, W.T.; Sabharwal, N.; Schneider, J.E.; Karamitsos, T.D.; et al. Relationship Between Left Ventricular Structural and Metabolic Remodeling in Type 2 Diabetes. *Diabetes* **2016**, *65*, 44–52. [CrossRef] [PubMed]
28. Jankovic, D.; Winhofer, Y.; Promintzer-Schifferl, M.; Wohlschläger-Krenn, E.; Anderwald, C.H.; Wolf, P.; Scherer, T.; Reiter, G.; Trattnig, S.; Luger, A.; et al. Effects of Insulin Therapy on Myocardial Lipid Content and Cardiac Geometry in Patients with Type-2 Diabetes Mellitus. *PLoS ONE* **2012**, *7*, e50077. [CrossRef] [PubMed]
29. Shah, R.V.; Abbasi, S.A.; Heydari, B.; Rickers, C.; Jacobs, D.R., Jr.; Wang, L.; Kwong, R.W.; Bluemke, D.A.; Lima, J.A.C.; Jerosch-Herold, M. Insulin resistance, subclinical left ventricular remodeling, and the obesity paradox: MESA (Multi-Ethnic Study of Atherosclerosis). *J. Am. Coll. Cardiol.* **2013**, *61*, 1698–1706. [CrossRef]
30. Packer, M. Differential Pathophysiological Mechanisms in Heart Failure with a Reduced or Preserved Ejection Fraction in Diabetes. *JACC Heart Fail.* **2021**, *9*, 535–549. [CrossRef]
31. Hasegawa, H.; Komuro, I. CHARM study-new strategy for the treatment of heart failure. *Nihon Rinsho. Jpn. J. Clin. Med.* **2004**, *62*, 995–1002.
32. Digitalis Investigation Group. The effect of digoxin on mortality and morbidity in patients with heart failure. *N. Engl. J. Med.* **1997**, *336*, 525–533. [CrossRef] [PubMed]
33. Massie, B.M.; Carson, P.E.; McMurray, J.J.; Komajda, M.; McKelvie, R.; Zile, M.R.; Andresen, S.; Donovan, M.; Iverson, E.; Staiger, C.; et al. Irbesartan in patients with heart failure and preserved ejection fraction. *N. Engl. J. Med.* **2008**, *359*, 2456–2467. [CrossRef]
34. Lindman, B.R.; Davila-Roman, V.G.; Mann, D.L.; McNulty, S.; Semigran, M.J.; Lewis, G.D.; de la Fuentes, L.; Vader, J.; Hernanderz, A.H.; Redfield, M.M.; et al. Cardiovascular phenotype in HFpEF patients with or without diabetes: A RELAX trial ancillary study. *J. Am. Coll. Cardiol.* **2014**, *64*, 541–549. [CrossRef]
35. Bellavite, P.; Fazio, S.; Affuso, F. A Descriptive Review of the Action Mechanisms of Berberine, Quercetin and Silymarin on Insulin Resistance/Hyperinsulinemia and Cardiovascular Prevention. *Molecules* **2023**, *28*, 4491. [CrossRef] [PubMed]
36. Redfield, M.M.; Chen, H.H.; Borlaug, B.A.; Semigran, M.J.; Lee, K.L.; Lewis, G.; Braunwald, E.; Anstrom, K.J.; Hernanderz, A.H.; O'Connor, C.M.; et al. Effect of phosphodiesterase-5 inhibition on exercise capacity and clinical status in heart failure with preserved ejection fraction: A randomized clinical trial. *JAMA* **2013**, *309*, 1268–1277. [CrossRef] [PubMed]
37. Yang, C.D.; Pan, W.Q.; Feng, S.; Quan, J.W.; Chen, J.W.; Shu, X.Y.; Aihemaiti, M.; Ding, F.H.; Shen, W.F.; Lu, L.; et al. Insulin Resistance Is Associated with Heart Failure with Recovered Ejection Fraction in Patients Without Diabetes. *J. Am. Heart Assoc.* **2022**, *11*, e026184. [CrossRef] [PubMed]
38. Jurczewska, J.; Ostrowska, J.; Che'chowska, M.; Panczyk, M.; Rudnicka, E.; Kucharski, M.; Smolarczyk, R.; Szostak-Węgierek, D. Physical activity, rather than diet, is linked to lower insulin resistance in PCOS women—A case control study. *Nutrients* **2023**, *15*, 2011. [CrossRef]
39. American Diabetes Association. Classification and Diagnosis of Diabetes: Standards of Medical Care in Diabetes—2020. *Diabetes Care* **2020**, *43* (Suppl. S1), S14–S31. [CrossRef]
40. Lopaschuk, G.D.; Karwi, Q.G.; Pherwani, S.; Ketema, E.B. Ketone metabolism in the failing heart. *Biochim. Biophys. Acta Mol. Cell Biol. Lipids* **2020**, *1865*, 158813. [CrossRef]
41. Hshemlu, L.; Esmaeili, R.; Bahramnezhad, F.; Rohani, C. A systematic review on clinical guidelines of nome health care in heart failure patients. *BMC Nurs.* **2023**, *22*, 127.
42. Butler, J.; Usman, M.S.; Khan, M.S.; Greene, S.J.; Friede, T.; Vaduganathan, M.; Filippatos, G.; Coats, A.J.S.; Anker, S.D. Efficacy and safety of SGLT2 inhibitors in heart failure: Systematic review and meta-analysis. *ESC Heart Fail.* **2020**, *7*, 3298–3309. [CrossRef]
43. Solomon, S.D.; McMurray, J.J.V.; Claggett, B.; de Boer, R.A.; De Mets, D.; Hernandez, A.F.; Inzucchi, S.E.; Kosiborod, M.N.; Lam, C.S.P.; Shah, S.J.; et al. Dapagliflozin in Heart Failure with Mildly Reduced or Preserved Ejection Fraction. *N. Engl. J. Med.* **2022**, *387*, 1089–1098. [CrossRef] [PubMed]
44. Vaduganathan, M.; Docherty, K.F.; Claggett, B.L.; Jhund, P.S.; de Boer, R.A.; Hernandez, A.F.; Inzucchi, S.E.; Kosiborod, M.N.; Lam, C.S.P.; Martinez, F.; et al. SGLT2 inhibitors in patients with heart failure: A comprehensive meta-analysis of five randomised controlled trials. *Lancet* **2022**, *400*, 757–767. [CrossRef]
45. Pabel, S.; Hamdani, N.; Luedde, M.; Sossalla, S. SGLT2 Inhibitors and Their Mode of Action in Heart Failure-Has the Mystery Been Unravelled? *Curr. Heart Fail Rep.* **2021**, *18*, 315–328. [CrossRef]
46. Hosokawa, Y.; Ogawa, W. SGLT2 inhibitors for genetic and acquired insulin resistance: Considerations for clinical use. *J. Diabetes Investig.* **2020**, *11*, 1431–1433. [CrossRef] [PubMed]
47. Salah, H.M.; Verma, S.; Santos-Gallego, C.G.; Bhatt, A.S.; Vaduganathan, M.; Khan, M.S.; Lopes, R.D.; Al'aref, S.J.; McGuire, D.K.; Fudim, M. Sodium-Glucose Cotransporter 2 Inhibitors and Cardiac Remodeling. *J. Cardiovasc. Transl. Res.* **2022**, *15*, 944–956. [CrossRef] [PubMed]
48. Dhingra, N.K.; Mistry, N.; Puar, P.; Verma, R.; Anker, S.; Mazer, C.D.; Verma, S. SGLT2 inhibitors and cardiac remodelling: A systematic review and meta-analysis of randomized cardiac magnetic resonance imaging trials. *ESC Heart Fail.* **2021**, *8*, 4693–4700. [CrossRef] [PubMed]
49. Song, X.-T.; Wei, Y.-L.; Rui, Y.-F.; Fan, L. Echocardiographic evaluation of the effect of dapagliflozin on epicardial adipose tissue and left ventricular systolic function in type 2 diabetes mellitus. *J. Diabetes Complicat.* **2023**, *37*, 108509. [CrossRef] [PubMed]

50. Bragazzi, N.L.; Zhong, W.; Shu, J.; Abu Much, A.; Lotan, D.; Grupper, A.; Younis, A.; Dai, H. Burden of heart failure and underlying causes in 195 countries and territories from 1990 to 2017. *Eur. J. Prev. Cardiol.* **2021**, *28*, 1682–1690. [CrossRef]
51. Halabi, A.; Sen, J.; Huynh, Q.; Marwick, T.H. Metformin treatment in heart failure with preserved ejection fraction: A systematic review and meta-regression analysis. *Cardiovasc. Diabetol.* **2020**, *19*, 124. [CrossRef]
52. Salvatore, T.; Galiero, R.; Caturano, A.; Vetrano, E.; Rinaldi, L.; Coviello, F.; Di Martino, A.; Albanese, G.; Marfella, R.; Sardu, C.; et al. Effects of Metformin in Heart Failure: From Pathophysiological Rationale to Clinical Evidence. *Biomolecules* **2021**, *11*, 1834. [CrossRef] [PubMed]
53. García, N.; Zazueta, C.; Aguilera-Aguirre, L. Oxidative Stress and Inflammation in Cardiovascular Disease. *Oxidative Med. Cell. Longev.* **2017**, *2017*, 5853238. [CrossRef] [PubMed]
54. Kamel, A.M.; Sabry, N.; Farid, S. Effect of metformin on left ventricular mass and functional parameters in non-diabetic patients: A meta-analysis of randomized clinical trials. *BMC Cardiovasc. Disord.* **2022**, *22*, 405. [CrossRef] [PubMed]
55. Wong, A.K.; Symon, R.; AlZadjali, M.A.; Ang, D.S.; Ogston, S.; Choy, A.; Petrie, J.R.; Struthers, A.D.; Lang, C.C. The effect of metformin on insulin resistance and exercise parameters in patients with heart failure. *Eur. J. Heart Fail.* **2012**, *14*, 1303–1310. [CrossRef] [PubMed]
56. Shen, Y.; Zhang, X.; Ma, W.; Song, H.; Gong, Z.; Wang, Q.; Che, L.; Xu, W.; Jiang, J.; Xu, J.; et al. VE/VCO2 slope and its prognostic value in patients with chronic heart failure. *Exp. Ther. Med.* **2015**, *9*, 1407–1412. [CrossRef] [PubMed]
57. Dagher, O.; Mury, P.; Thorin-Trescases, N.; Noly, P.E.; Thorin, E.; Carrier, M. Therapeutic Potential of Quercetin to Alleviate Endothelial Dysfunction in Age-Related Cardiovascular Diseases. *Front. Cardiovasc. Med.* **2021**, *8*, 658400. [CrossRef]
58. Tamtaji, O.R.; Milajerdi, A.; Dadgostar, E.; Kolahdooz, F.; Chamani, M.; Amirani, E.; Mirzaei, H.; Asemi, Z. The Effects of Quercetin Supplementation on Blood Pressures and Endothelial Function Among Patients with Metabolic Syndrome and Related Disorders: A Systematic Review and Meta-analysis of Randomized Controlled Trials. *Curr. Pharm. Des.* **2019**, *25*, 1372–1384. [CrossRef]
59. Hosseini, A.; Razavi, B.M.; Banach, M.; Hosseinzadeh, H. Quercetin and metabolic syndrome: A review. *Phytotherapy Res.* **2021**, *35*, 5352–5364. [CrossRef] [PubMed]
60. Li, X.; Wang, R.; Zhou, N.; Wang, X.; Liu, Q.; Bai, Y.; Bai, Y.; Liu, Z.; Yang, H.; Zou, J.; et al. Quercetin improves insulin resistance and hepatic lipid accumulation in vitro in a NAFLD cell model. *Biomed. Rep.* **2013**, *1*, 71–76. [CrossRef]
61. Kang, J.S.; Jeon, Y.J.; Kim, H.M.; Han, S.H.; Yang, K.-H. Inhibition of Inducible Nitric-Oxide Synthase Expression by Silymarin in Lipopolysaccharide-Stimulated Macrophages. *J. Pharmacol. Exp. Ther.* **2002**, *302*, 138–144. [CrossRef]
62. Guo, Y.; Wang, S.; Wang, Y.; Zhu, T. Silymarin improved diet-induced liver damage and insulin resistance by decreasing inflammation in mice. *Pharm. Biol.* **2016**, *54*, 2995–3000. [CrossRef] [PubMed]
63. Feng, B.; Huang, B.; Jing, Y.; Shen, S.; Feng, W.; Wang, W.; Meng, R.; Zhu, D. Silymarin ameliorates the disordered glucose metabolism of mice with diet-induced obesity by activating the hepatic SIRT1 pathway. *Cell. Signal.* **2021**, *84*, 110023. [CrossRef] [PubMed]
64. Li, H.B.; Yang, Y.R.; Mo, Z.J.; Ding, Y.; Jiang, W.J. Silibinin improves palmitate-induced insulin resistance in C2C12 myotubes by attenuating IRS-1/PI3K/Akt pathway inhibition. *Braz. J. Med. Biol. Res.* **2015**, *48*, 440–446. [CrossRef] [PubMed]
65. Bouderba, S.; Sanchez-Martin, C.; Villanueva, G.R.; Detaille, D.; Koceïr, E.A. Beneficial effects of silibinin against the progression of metabolic syndrome, increased oxidative stress, and liver steatosis in *Psammomys obesus*, a relevant animal model of human obesity and diabetes. *J. Diabetes* **2014**, *6*, 184–192. [CrossRef]
66. Zeng, X.-H.; Li, Y.-Y. Efficacy and safety of berberine for congestive heart failure secondary to ischemic or idiopathic dilated cardiomyopathy. *Am. J. Cardiol.* **2003**, *92*, 173–176. [CrossRef] [PubMed]
67. Zeng, X.; Zeng, X. Relationship between the clinical effects of berberine on severe congestive heart failure and its concentration in plasma studied by HPLC. *Biomed. Chromatogr.* **1999**, *13*, 442–444. [CrossRef]
68. Carlomagno, G.; Affuso, F.; Napoli, R.; Mercurio, V.; Fazio, V.; Micillo, F.; Pirozzi, C.; Ruvolo, A.; Saccá, L.; Fazio, S. A nutraceutical combination improves insulin sensitivity in patients with metabolic syndrome. *World J. Cardiol.* **2012**, *4*, 77–83. [CrossRef]
69. Mercurio, V.; Pucci, G.; Bosso, G.; Fazio, V.; Battista, F.; Iannuzzi, A.; Brambilla, N.; Vitalini, C.; D'Amato, M.; Giacovelli, G.; et al. A nutraceutical combination reduces left ventricular mass in subjects with metabolic syndrome and left ventricular hypertrophy: A multicenter, randomized, double-blind, placebo-controlled trial. *Clin. Nutr.* **2020**, *39*, 1379–1384. [CrossRef]
70. Muller, T.D.; Finan, B.; Bloom, S.R.; D'Alessio, D.; Drucker, D.J.; Flatt, P.R.; Fritsche, A.; Gribble, F.; Grill, H.J.; Habener, J.F.; et al. Glucagon-lime peptide 1 (GLP-1). *Mol. Metab.* **2019**, *30*, 72–130. [CrossRef]
71. Ferreira, J.P.; Saraiva, F.; Sharma, A.; Vasques-Nóvoa, F.; Angélico-Gonçalves, A.; Leite, A.R.; Borges-Canha, M.; Carvalho, D.; Packer, M.; Zannad, F.; et al. Glucagon-like peptide 1 receptor agonists in patients with type 2 diabetes with and without chronic heart failure: A meta-analysis of randomized placebo-controlled outcome trials. *Diabetes Obes. Metab.* **2023**, *25*, 1495–1502. [CrossRef]
72. Merza, N.; Akram, M.; Mengal, A.; Rashid, A.M.; Mahboob, A.; Faryad, M.; Fatima, Z.; Ahmed, M.; Ansari, S.A. The Safety and Efficacy of GLP-1 Receptor Agonists in Heart Failure Patients: A Systematic Review and Meta-Analysis. *Curr. Probl. Cardiol.* **2023**, *48*, 101602. [CrossRef] [PubMed]
73. Wicklmayr, M.; Rett, K.; Dietze, G.; Mehnert, H. Effects of beta-blocking agents on insulin secretion and glucose disposal. *Horm. Metab. Res. Suppl.* **1990**, *22*, 29–33. [PubMed]

74. Jacob, S. Beta-blocking agents in patients with insulin resistance: Effects of vasodilating beta-blockers. *Blood Press* **1999**, *8*, 261–268. [CrossRef]
75. Buscemi, S.; Nicolucci, A.; Lucisano, G.; Galvano, F.; Grosso, G.; Massenti, F.M.; Amodio, E.; Bonura, A.; Sprini, D.; Rini, G.B. Impact of chronic diuretic treatment on glucose homeostasis. *Diabetol. Metab. Syndr.* **2013**, *5*, 80. [CrossRef]
76. Ramsay, L.E.; Yeo, W.W.; Jackson, P.R. Diabetes, impaired glucose tolerance and insulin resistance with diuretics. *Eur. Heart J.* **1992**, *13*, 68–71. [CrossRef]
77. Dronavalli, S.; Bakris, G.L.; Kaplan, N.M.; Raheja, P.; Price, A.; Wang, Z.; Arbique, D.; Adams-Huet, B.; Auchus, R.J.; Vongpatanasin, W.; et al. Mechanistic Insights into Diuretic-Induced Insulin Resistance. *Hypertension* **2008**, *52*, 1009–1011. [CrossRef] [PubMed]
78. Abbasi, F.; Lamendola, C.; Harris, C.S.; Harris, V.; Tsai, M.-S.; Tripathi, P.; Abbas, F.; Reaven, G.M.; Reaven, P.D.; Snyder, M.P.; et al. Statins Are Associated with Increased Insulin Resistance and Secretion. *Arter. Thromb. Vasc. Biol.* **2021**, *41*, 2786–2797. [CrossRef]

biomedicines

MDPI

Article

Association between Serum Free Fatty Acids and Clinical and Laboratory Parameters in Acute Heart Failure Patients

Iva Klobučar [1], Helga Hinteregger [2], Margarete Lechleitner [2], Matias Trbušić [1,3], Gudrun Pregartner [4], Andrea Berghold [4], Wolfgang Sattler [2,5], Saša Frank [2,5,*] and Vesna Degoricija [3,6]

1 Department of Cardiology, Sisters of Charity University Hospital Centre, 10000 Zagreb, Croatia; iva.klobucar@gmail.com (I.K.); matias.trbusic@gmail.com (M.T.)
2 Gottfried Schatz Research Center, Molecular Biology and Biochemistry, Medical University of Graz, 8010 Graz, Austria; helga.reicher@medunigraz.at (H.H.); margarete.lechleitner@medunigraz.at (M.L.); wolfgang.sattler@medunigraz.at (W.S.)
3 School of Medicine, University of Zagreb, 10000 Zagreb, Croatia; vesna.degoricija@mef.hr
4 Institute for Medical Informatics, Statistics and Documentation, Medical University of Graz, 8036 Graz, Austria; gudrun.pregartner@medunigraz.at (G.P.); andrea.berghold@medunigraz.at (A.B.)
5 BioTechMed-Graz, 8010 Graz, Austria
6 Department of Medicine, Sisters of Charity University Hospital Centre, 10000 Zagreb, Croatia
* Correspondence: sasa.frank@medunigraz.at; Tel.: +43-316-385-71969

Abstract: Very little is known about the association between individual serum free fatty acids (FFAs) and clinical and laboratory parameters (indicators of heart failure severity) in acute heart failure (AHF) patients. Here, the baseline serum levels of FFAs, 16:0 (palmitic acid), 16:1 (palmitoleic acid), 18:0 (stearic acid), 18:1 (oleic acid), 18:2 (linoleic acid), 18:3 (alpha-linolenic acid or gamma-linolenic acid), 20:4 (arachidonic acid), 20:5 (eicosapentaenoic acid), and 22:6 (docosahexaenoic acid), were determined in 304 AHF patients (94.7% belonged to New York Heart Association functional class IV) using gas chromatography. Spearman correlation coefficients were used to examine the associations between the individual and total (the sum of all FFAs) FFAs and clinical and laboratory parameters. After applying a Bonferroni correction to correct for multiple testing, the total FFAs, as well as the individual FFAs (except FFAs 18:0, 20:5, and 22:6), were found to be significantly positively correlated with serum albumin. Only a few additional associations were found: FFA 16:0 was significantly negatively correlated with systolic pulmonary artery pressure, FFA 18:3 was significantly negatively correlated with C-reactive protein and body mass index, and FFA 20:4 was significantly negatively correlated with blood urea nitrogen. Based on our results, we conclude that in patients with severe AHF, individual and total serum FFAs are slightly associated with established laboratory and clinical parameters, which are indicators of heart failure severity.

Keywords: acute heart failure; free fatty acids; gas chromatography

1. Introduction

Heart failure (HF) is the final stage of various cardiovascular diseases and therefore a frequent cause of disability and death worldwide [1]. The failing heart exhibits an altered structure and consequently an impaired function, resulting in the diminished perfusion of metabolizing tissues [2–4]. Acute heart failure (AHF) is characterized by either the rapid onset or worsening of the signs and symptoms of HF [3].

Decreased peripheral perfusion in HF triggers compensatory mechanisms, which then further deteriorate the underlying pathophysiology, leading to disease progression and increased severity [5]. More specifically, the under-perfusion of kidneys stimulates the renin–angiotensin system (RAS) and, in turn, aldosterone and norepinephrine secretion. This leads to increased renal sodium and water retention, as well as increased systemic blood pressure, which further weakens the function of the failing heart [6]. Left ventricular dysfunction and heart wall distension trigger an elevation in natriuretic peptides, which only partially counteract the effects of activated RAS, aldosterone, and increased sympathetic tone. Peripheral venous congestion (a consequence of right-sided HF) and hypoperfusion worsen renal and liver function and also diminish the motility of the gut, resulting in an altered composition of the gut microbiota and leading to gut inflammation and diminished nutrient absorption, as well as a systemic inflammatory response [7–10]. The latter is primarily caused by the compromised barrier function of the edematous and inflamed intestine and consequently the increased translocation of bacterial toxins into the circulation, as well as the congestion-induced activation of venous endothelial cells [11,12].

Increased serum levels of catecholamines, natriuretic peptides, and inflammatory cytokines are strong inducers of adipose tissue lipolysis, the hallmark of catabolic dominance and a major source of serum free fatty acids (FFAs) [13,14]. Serum FFAs are also generated by the serum-lipase-mediated hydrolysis of lipids in circulating lipoproteins, a process regulated by nutritional state, hormones, and inflammatory cytokines [15]. High serum levels of FFAs are potent inducers of insulin resistance, a frequent pathophysiological component of HF, as well as oxidative stress, inflammatory response, and endothelial dysfunction, with the latter being an inherent feature of vascular pathophysiology in HF [16–18]. In HF, an increased uptake of FFAs by cardiomyocytes, secondary to elevated FFA serum levels, leads to the accumulation of FFA-derived cardiotoxic intermediates that, together with diminished glucose and increased FFA utilization for cardiac ATP production, deteriorate the function of the failing heart [19–21]. Pharmacological interventions capable of reducing FFAs and increasing glucose utilization for energy production improve cardiac function and prognosis in patients with chronic HF (CHF) [18,22–24].

Total serum FFA levels are higher in patients with CHF compared with healthy controls, and high levels of total FFAs have been found to be associated with increased mortality in AHF patients [25–27]. Several studies have examined the association between various individual serum FFAs and mortality in AHF patients [28–31], but none of them have reported on the association of studied FFAs with patients' clinical and laboratory characteristics. Therefore, in the present study, we determined the serum levels of FFAs 16:0 (palmitic acid), 16:1 (palmitoleic acid), 18:0 (stearic acid), 18:1 (oleic acid), 18:2 (linoleic acid), 18:3 (alpha-linolenic acid or gamma-linolenic acid), 20:4 (arachidonic acid), 20:5 (eicosapentaenoic acid), and 22:6 (docosahexaenoic acid) and examined their association with clinical and laboratory parameters, established indicators of HF severity, in AHF patients.

2. Materials and Methods

2.1. Study Design and Patients

The AHF study was a prospective observational study conducted at the Sisters of Charity University Hospital Centre, Zagreb, Croatia, from March 2018 to January 2021, enrolling consecutive adult Caucasian patients who presented to the Emergency Department with signs and symptoms of AHF consequently requiring hospitalization. The coexistence of any case of acute infection, chronic obstructive pulmonary disease exacerbation, severe renal failure (creatinine serum levels of >400 μmol/L), active malignant disease, systemic autoimmune disease, pregnancy, or a patient's unwillingness to participate led to their exclusion from the study (study flow chart—Scheme S1). Details from the data collection on the patients' history as well as physical and echocardiography examinations were described in our previous reports [32,33]. In addition to routinely performed laboratory tests, for study purposes, a sample of 36 mL of venous blood was obtained from each study patient at the time they presented to the Emergency Department. All enrolled patients received guideline-directed treatment for AHF, as proposed by the European Society of Cardiology [4]. Study patients were followed up for one year after index AHF hospitalization, and the primary endpoint was all-cause mortality.

Prior to enrolment and any study procedure, written informed consent for participation was obtained from each enrolled patient in compliance with the Good Clinical Practice guidelines, and the investigation conformed with the principles outlined in the Declaration of Helsinki [34]. The study was approved by the local Ethics Committee of the Sisters of Charity University Hospital Centre, Zagreb, Croatia (EP 2258/18-10), and the Medical University of Graz, Austria (EK 33-258 ex 20/21).

2.2. Laboratory Analyses and Procedures

Routine laboratory parameters, assessed at the time of the patients' presentation to the Emergency Department, regardless of their fasting status as per hospital protocols for AHF management, included creatinine, estimated glomerular filtration rate (eGFR), blood urea nitrogen, sodium, potassium, chloride, serum glucose, total protein, albumin, total cholesterol, high-density lipoprotein cholesterol (HDL-C), low-density lipoprotein cholesterol (LDL-C), triglycerides, C-reactive protein (CRP), bilirubin, alanine aminotransferase (ALT), aspartate aminotransferase (AST), lactate dehydrogenase (LDH), creatine kinase (CK), high-sensitivity troponin I (hsTnI), N-terminal pro-brain natriuretic peptide (NT-proBNP), blood cell counts, and hemoglobin, fibrinogen, prothrombin time, and international normalized ratio (INR), as well as arterial blood gases. Laboratory procedures and equipment used for assessment of the abovementioned parameters have been described in detail in our previous reports [32]. All additional laboratory procedures and analyses for study purposes were performed using the stored samples of the patients' sera at the Gottfried Schatz Research Center, Medical University of Graz, Graz, Austria.

2.3. Quantification of FFAs

All solvents and reagents were from Sigma-Aldrich (St. Louis, MO, USA). To quantify FFAs, 190 μL of serum was subjected to a Folch extraction (4 mL of chloroform/methanol at 2:1 ratio and 2 mL of water) on a rotating wheel (45 min at ambient temperature). Samples were then centrifuged (500× *g*, 10 min, 4 °C), the lower phase was removed, and the aqueous phase was reextracted. The organic phases were combined, dried under a stream of N_2, transferred to autosampler vials, and stored under argon at −80 °C. To isolate serum FFAs, the total lipid fraction was subjected to thin-layer chromatography (TLC, unmodified Silica Gel 60 (Merck, Darmstadt, Germany) developed in hexane/diethylether/acetic acid; 70:30:1. The silica region comigrating with oleic acid (spotted on one lane as the FFA standard, stained with iodine vapor) was scraped off, transferred to conical screw-capped derivatization vials, spiked with pentadecanoic acid (C15; 10 μg of internal standard for GC quantitation), and directly methylated (toluene, 1.2 mL; boron trifluoride/methanol complex, 20%; 1 mL; 60 min at 110 °C, sand bath) in the presence of the TLC adsorbent. The reaction was stopped with water (2 mL); fatty acid methyl esters (FAMEs) were extracted with hexane (200 μL), transferred to autosampler vials, dried under N_2, and redissolved in toluene (25 μL). The FAMEs (1 μL) were analyzed on a Thermo Trace GC Ultra gas chromatograph (Thermo Fisher Scientific, Vienna, Austria) with flame ionization detection (FID). Samples were separated on a 25 m × 0.32 mm FFAP-CB column (Agilent, Vienna, Austria) using the following GC conditions: injector 230 °C, detector 250 °C, with ramping starting at 150 °C, 2.5 °C/min, 215 °C, 10 min, 10 °C/min, and 230 °C, 12.5 min. Fatty acid concentrations were quantified via peak area comparison with the internal standard (C15) and converted to μmol/L. FAMEs prepared from a control serum were run after every 23rd patient sample (the daily throughput) as a laboratory control sample.

2.4. Statistics

Metric parameters are summarized as the mean and standard deviation (SD) or median and interquartile range, whereas absolute and relative frequencies were used to describe categorical parameters. Differences between groups defined by various clinical characteristics were tested with the Mann–Whitney U test. The Spearman correlation coefficient was used to assess correlations between FFAs and various clinical and laboratory parameters. Results are presented in a heatmap. A p-value < 0.005 (0.05/10) was considered significant after a Bonferroni correction for multiple testing due to the 10 investigated FFA parameters. Our data allow for the detection of significant group differences between alive and deceased patients within 12 months (n = 190 vs. n = 114) for effect sizes of at least 0.39 or for correlation coefficients within the whole cohort (n = 304) of at least 0.19, with a power of 90%. R version 4.1.0 was used for these analyses.

3. Results

3.1. Patients' Clinical Characteristics, Chronic Medication, and Standard Laboratory Parameters

A total of 315 patients hospitalized due to AHF were enrolled in the study. The baseline characteristics, comorbidities, chronic medication, and routine laboratory parameters of the whole cohort have been described in our previous reports [32,33].

Since not all serum samples were available for FFA quantification, the following analyses and presented results are based on the data collected from 304 participants.

The patients' mean (±standard deviation) age was 74.3 ± 10.5 years, and 131 (43.1%) were female. As 281 (92.4%) patients suffered from previously known cardiomyopathy (secondary ischemic, valvular, toxic etiology, primary dilated cardiomyopathies), their present episode of AHF was classified as worsening of chronic disease, while only 23 (7.6%) patients presented with new-onset AHF. The dominant cause of the new-onset AHF was acute myocardial infarction (17/23, 73.9%; 11 with anteroseptal localization and 6 with inferoposterior/posterolateral localization). Only three (1.0%) of the enrolled patients suffered from isolated right ventricle failure (after disqualification of participation for dyspneic patients with chronic pulmonary diseases), while the rest (301, 99.0%) had signs and symptoms of left-sided or global (combination of left- and right-sided) HF. Of the latter, 55 patients (18.3%) presented with pulmonary edema (out of which 60% were hypertensive forms), while the remaining 246 (81.7%) patients with left-sided or global HF had less severe signs of lung congestion. Four patients (1.3%) suffered from cardiogenic shock at the time of presentation to the Emergency Department. According to NYHA classification, the majority of the enrolled patients (288, 94.7%) had dyspnea and tachypnea at rest (NYHA IV), while the others (16, 5.3%) were asymptomatic at rest but could not tolerate minimal physical effort (NYHA III) at the time of presentation. The patients' comorbidities, vital signs, and other clinical signs of HF, as well as significant echocardiographic measures and routine laboratory test results obtained at the time of presentation to the Emergency Department, are shown in Table 1. Chronic medication is listed in Table S1. One hundred and fourteen (37.5%) patients died within one year after index AHF hospitalization.

Table 1. Baseline characteristics and laboratory data of AHF patients.

	Data For All Patients with FFA (n = 304)
Demographics	
Age (years)	74.3 (10.5)
Sex, female	131 (43.1%)
Comorbidities	
Hypertension	283 (93.1%)
T2DM	128 (42.1%)
CAD	152 (50.0%)
CMP	281 (92.4%)
AF	167 (54.9%)
CKD	139 (45.7%)
MetS	208 (68.4%)
Physical measures at admission	
MAP (mmHg)	100.0 (90.0, 118.8)

Table 1. *Cont.*

	Data For All Patients with FFA (n = 304)
Heart rate (beats/min)	100.0 (80.0, 115.5)
Respiratory rate (breaths/min)	28.0 (24.0, 32.5)
BMI (kg/m^2)	28.0 (25.0, 31.7)
Signs and symptoms	
Symptom duration (days)	5.0 (4.0, 5.0)
Rales or crackles	300 (98.7%)
JVD	165 (54.3%)
Enlarged liver	171 (56.2%)
Ascites	47 (15.5%)
Peripheral edema	198 (65.1%)
NYHA class	
3	16 (5.3%)
4	288 (94.7%)
AHF type	
New-onset AHF	23 (7.6%)
AHF following CHF	281 (92.4%)
Echocardiography	
LVEDd/BSA (mm/m^2)	28.6 (25.5, 31.8)
LVEF (%)	40.0 (30.0, 50.0)
SPAP (mmHg)	50.0 (45.0, 60.0)
AHF class	
HFrEF, EF < 40%	138 (47.1%)
HFmrEF, EF 41-49%	80 (27.3%)
HFpEF, EF ≥ 50%	75 (25.6%)
Laboratory test results at admission	
TC (mmol/L)	3.5 (2.9, 4.5)
HDL-C (mmol/L)	1.1 (0.9, 1.3)
LDL-C (mmol/L)	1.9 (1.4, 2.7)
Triglycerides (mmol/L)	1.0 (0.8, 1.3)
Albumin (g/L)	37.9 (34.9, 41.3)
Total proteins (g/L)	67.0 (61.0, 71.0)
Bilirubin (μmol/L)	17.3 (11.2, 28.5)
AST (U/L)	27.0 (20.0, 44.2)
ALT (U/L)	25.0 (15.0, 41.2)
Glucose (mmol/L)	7.8 (6.1, 11.1)
Sodium (mmol/L)	140.0 (137.0, 142.0)
Potassium (mmol/L)	4.5 (4.1, 4.8)
Chloride (mmol/L)	103.0 (99.0, 106.0)
BUN (mmol/L)	9.6 (7.0, 14.1)
Creatinine (μmol/L)	117.0 (89.8, 152.0)
eGFR (mL/min/1.73m^2)	46.3 (32.4, 64.3)
CK (U/L)	93.5 (58.0, 162.2)
LDH (U/L)	264.0 (218.8, 329.2)
hsTnI (ng/L)	46.0 (20.0, 141.0)

Table 1. *Cont.*

	Data For All Patients with FFA (n = 304)
NT-proBNP (pg/mL)	6578.5 (3544.5, 15076.2)
CRP (mg/L)	11.8 (5.5, 32.6)
IL-6 (pg/mL)	25.1 (12.9, 59.8)
Fibrinogen (g/L)	4.0 (3.4, 4.7)
Erythrocytes (x 10^{12}/L)	4.6 (4.1, 5.0)
Hemoglobin (g/L)	133.5 (119.0, 148.0)
pH	7.4 (7.3, 7.4)
pO_2 (kPa)	8.8 (7.3, 10.4)
pCO_2 (kPa)	5.2 (4.5, 6.4)
HCO_3 (mmol/L)	24.0 (21.3, 27.5)

Data are presented as n (%), mean and standard deviation, or as median and interquartile range (q1, q3). AF, atrial fibrillation; AHF, acute heart failure; ALT, alanine aminotransferase; AST, aspartate aminotransferase; BMI, body mass index; BUN, blood urea nitrogen; CAD, coronary artery disease; CHF, chronic heart failure; CK, creatine kinase; CKD, chronic kidney disease; CMP, cardiomyopathy; CRP, C-reactive protein; EF, ejection fraction; eGFR, estimated glomerular filtration rate; HDL-C, high-density lipoprotein cholesterol; HFrEF, heart failure with reduced ejection fraction; HFmrEF, heart failure with mildly reduced ejection fraction; HFpEF, heart failure with preserved ejection fraction; hsTnI, high-sensitivity troponin I; HDL-C, high-density lipoprotein cholesterol; JVD, jugular vein distension; LDH, lactate dehydrogenase; LDL-C, low-density lipoprotein cholesterol; LVEDd, left ventricle end-diastolic diameter; LVEF, left ventricular ejection fraction; MAP, mean arterial pressure; MetS, metabolic syndrome; NT-proBNP, N-terminal pro-brain natriuretic peptide; NYHA, New York Heart Association Functional Classification; pO_2, partial oxygen pressure; pCO_2, partial carbon dioxide pressure; SPAP, systolic pulmonary artery pressure; TC, total cholesterol; T2DM, diabetes mellitus type 2.

3.2. Levels of FFAs in Serum of AHF Patients

We determined the concentrations of nine individual FFAs and the sum of these in the serum of 304 AHF patients. The most abundant FFAs were 18:1, 16:0, 18:2, and 18:0. Markedly lower concentrations were found for FFA 16:1, followed by 20:4 and 18:3, whereas the lowest concentrations were found for FFAs 22:6 and 20:5 (Table 2).

Table 2. FFA levels in AHF patients (N = 304).

FFA	Serum Levels (µmol/L)
16:0	260.5 (195.9, 310.6)
16:1	25.9 (15.9, 39.8)
18:0	122.8 (97.9, 153.9)
18:1	304.6 (221.8, 404.9)
18:2	150.5 (100.8, 203.6)
18:3	5.1 (3.5, 7.7)
20:4	7.2 (5.3, 10.6)
20:5	0.3 (0.2, 0.7)
22:6	1.2 (0.8, 1.7)
Sum	896.8 (667.3, 1126.2)

Data are presented as median and interquartile range (q1, q3). FFA, free fatty acid.

3.3. Associations of Serum FFAs with Clinical and Laboratory Parameters in AHF Patients

As shown in Figure 1, after a Bonferroni correction for multiple testing, the individual FFAs 16:0, 16:1, 18:1, 18:2, 18:3, and 20:4, as well as the total FFAs, were significantly positively correlated with serum albumin levels, albeit not very strongly. Additionally, FFA 16:0 was significantly negatively correlated with systolic pulmonary artery pressure (SPAP), and FFA 20:4 was significantly negatively correlated with blood urea nitrogen (BUN), whereas FFA 18:3 was significantly negatively correlated with C-reactive protein (CRP) and body mass index (BMI). We found no significant correlations of any individual FFA or total

FFAs with N-terminal pro-brain natriuretic peptide (NT-proBNP), left ventricular ejection fraction (LVEF), mean arterial pressure (MAP), hemoglobin, liver transaminases, creatine kinase (CK), glucose, creatinine, and estimated glomerular filtration rate (eGFR), as well as interleukin-6 (IL-6) and serum lipid parameters (Figure 1).

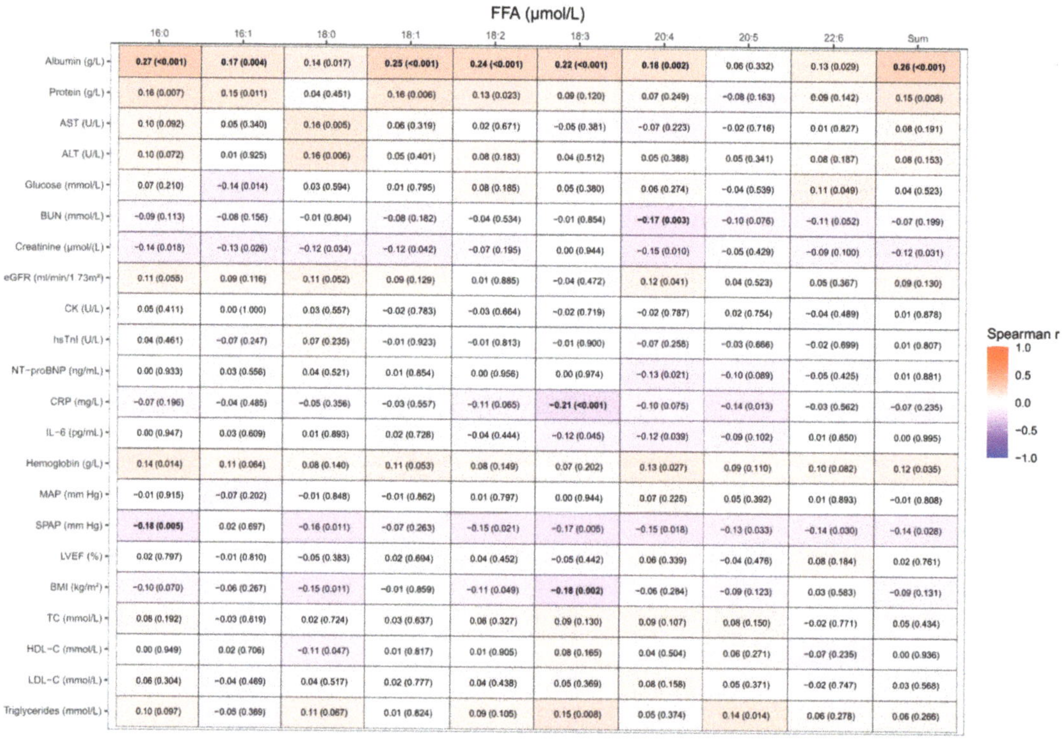

Figure 1. Heatmap of correlation analyses between FFA and the laboratory and clinical parameters of patients with AHF. Values presented are the Spearman correlation coefficients. p-values < 0.005 after a Bonferroni correction for multiple testing are considered significant, and significant correlations are depicted in bold. Albumin, protein, and LVEF were measured in 293 patients, SPAP was measured in 253 patients, BUN in 303, and hsTnI in 301 patients; otherwise, the analyses are based on 304 samples. ALT, alanine aminotransferase; AST, aspartate aminotransferase; BMI, body mass index; BUN, blood urea nitrogen; CK, creatin kinase; CRP, C-reactive protein; eGFR, estimated glomerular filtration rate; HDL-C, high-density lipoprotein cholesterol; hsTnI, high-sensitivity troponin I; IL-6, interleukin-6; LDL-C, low-density lipoprotein cholesterol; LVEF, left ventricular ejection fraction; MAP, mean arterial pressure; NT-proBNP, N-terminal pro-brain natriuretic peptide; SPAP, systolic pulmonary pressure; TC, total cholesterol.

3.4. Differences in FFAs in Various Groups of AHF Patients

We also examined whether the serum levels of individual and total FFAs differed in groups of AHF patients defined by various clinical characteristics and survival statuses. The results are shown in Tables S2 and S3. After Bonferroni correction, the serum levels of FFA 16:1 but not of the other individual or total FFAs were significantly lower in AHF patients with type 2 diabetes mellitus (T2D) and in AHF patients with coronary artery disease (CAD) compared with AHF patients without these comorbidities. In contrast, the serum levels of individual and total FFAs were similar in AHF patients with metabolic syndrome (MetS), atrial fibrillation (AF), and sign(s) of venous volume overload compared with AHF patients without these comorbidities or sign(s), as well as in AHF patients with new-onset AHF compared with those with AHF that developed on top of CHF. The serum levels of the individual and total FFAs were also similar in AHF patients who were alive and those who died during index AHF hospitalization or within 3 or 12 months after hospitalization due to AHF.

4. Discussion

Increased serum levels of natriuretic peptides, catecholamines, and inflammatory cytokines are major promoters of insulin resistance, catabolic dominance, and lipolysis in HF. High-circulating FFAs facilitate cardiac uptake and utilization of FFAs as energy substrates, as well as the conversion of FFAs into lipotoxic compounds [13,20,32]. Deranged cardiac energy metabolism and lipotoxicity compromise the contractile function of the failing heart [13,20,32]. In line with this, elevated total serum FFAs were associated with poor outcomes in AHF patients [26,27], and pharmacological inhibition of cardiac FFA utilization for energy production improved the cardiac function and reduced mortality in AHF patients [22,23].

In contrast to the total serum FFA levels, several studies reported a negative association of serum levels of various individual FFAs with mortality in AHF patients [28–31]. Low serum levels of FFAs may reflect low adipose tissue lipolysis, increased FFA consumption, or decreased supply due to malnutrition, which is highly prevalent in patients with AHF [33]. Reduced appetite and impaired intestinal absorption, due to gut inflammation, hypoperfusion, and congestion, together with low-grade persistent systemic inflammation, cause malnutrition, wasting, and frailty, the typical features of advanced HF, which are positively associated with unfavorable prognosis in HF patients [33,34].

In the present study, we determined the serum levels of nine individual FFAs and examined the associations of these individual and total FFAs with clinical and laboratory parameters in our AHF patients. In line with the well-established physiological role of albumin as a vehicle for the transport of hydrophobic FFAs, the serum levels of the majority of FFAs were significantly positively correlated with albumin. Since decreased serum albumin reflects a poor nutritional state, impaired intestinal absorption, and reduced biosynthetic capacity of the liver [35], the observed positive associations of FFAs with albumin may suggest a relationship between FFAs, nutritional state, and intestinal and liver function in AHF patients.

Additionally, we found a significant negative association of FFA 16:0 with SPAP and of FFA 20:4 with BUN. These negative associations most likely reflect the regulation of these FFAs, as well as that of SPAP and BUN, in the opposite direction by the underlying AHF pathophysiology. While the HF pathophysiology decreases FFAs levels via the promotion of malnutrition and wasting, the concomitantly worsened renal function (due to hypoperfusion and congestion) increases BUN [8,36], whereas the worsened left ventricular function and consequently increased left ventricular filling pressure increase SPAP [6,37]. Interestingly, these results suggest that FFAs 16:0 and 20:4 do not contribute to the postulated impairment of the heart contractility by toxic derivatives of FFAs in the environment with increased serum levels of FFAs [20]. Several other individual FFAs and the total FFAs were weakly negatively associated with SPAP; however, after a Bonferroni correction, these associations did not remain statistically significant. The significant negative association of FFA 18:3 with CRP that was observed in the present study is in accordance with an inverse association of dietary intake of FFA 18:3 with CRP, as described in a previous study [38]. Although numerous studies reported on the cardiovascular protective effects and anti-inflammatory activities of FFAs 20:5 and 22:6, these FFAs were not significantly associated with CRP or IL-6 in the present study [39,40]. In line with the reported negative association between various plasma FFAs with BMI (reviewed in [41]), in the present study, FFA 18:3 was significantly negatively associated with BMI. Metabolic constellations in adipose tissue and low-grade persistent inflammation have been shown to be potent modulators of desaturases and elongases, the enzymes which catalyze the conversion of FFA 18:3 into FFAs 20:5 and 22:6 [41]. Additionally, a higher BMI may be accompanied by a higher demand for FFAs as energy substrates or for their incorporation into lipids in various tissues, thus resulting in lower serum levels and negative associations of these FFAs with BMI. Several other individual FFAs also showed a weak negative association with BMI, although this did not reach statistical significance.

In the present study, in which 94.7% of patients belonged to New York Heart Association functional class IV (NYHA IV), total serum FFAs were neither associated (with exception of albumin) with clinical and laboratory parameters nor with mortality of these patients. This is in sharp contrast to the results obtained in other AHF cohorts in which the majority of patients belonged to NYHA class III and where total serum FFAs were significantly associated with several clinical and laboratory parameters, as well as mortality [26,27]. This implies that the pathophysiology in severe AHF, as encountered in NYHA class IV patients, disrupts the associations of serum FFAs with clinical and laboratory indicators of the HF severity, as well as abolishing the prognostic capacity of FFAs.

Previous studies have reported associations of circulating FFAs with various comorbidities associated with HF, such as T2D, CAD, hypertension, or AF [42–45]. In line with the reported beneficial effect of FFA 16:1 on insulin secretion and systemic insulin sensitivity [46], we observed higher FFA 16:1 serum levels in our AHF patients without T2D compared with those with this comorbidity. Higher FFA 16:1 levels in our AHF patients without CAD, compared with those with CAD, suggest a cardioprotective effect of this FFA. However, although FFA 16:1 has been shown to contribute to an anti-atherogenic serum lipoprotein profile, the impact of FFA 16:1 on the cardiovascular system is still not well understood [47].

It is well established that adipose tissue lipolysis mediated by the sequential action of adipose triglyceride lipase (ATGL), hormone-sensitive lipase, and monoglyceride lipase is essential for the supply of tissues with FFAs from the adipose triacylglycerol (TAG) pool to enable the maintenance of systemic energy metabolism during fasting or physical activity, the conditions accompanied by low circulating glucose levels and a high energy demand [48]. However, excessive activation of adipose tissue lipolysis secondary to increased adrenergic activation or increased serum levels of natriuretic peptides and inflammatory cytokines, as encountered in HF, leads to pathologically increased serum levels and increased tissue uptake of FFAs (reviewed in [49]). Excessive uptake and accumulation of TAG and lipotoxic intermediates in the liver and skeletal muscle activate specific protein kinase C isoforms, leading to impaired insulin signaling and T2D [50–52]. Insulin resistance in adipose tissue, which in HF is triggered by persistent low-grade inflammation, attenuates the antilipolytic action of insulin and thus also contributes to an increase in serum FFAs and systemic insulin resistance [53]. The impact of adipose-tissue-released FFAs on metabolic health was also demonstrated in obese mice in which adipose-tissue-specific genetic inactivation of ATGL, a master regulator of adipose tissue lipolysis, reduced plasma FFAs and hepatic lipid content, eventually resulting in an improved insulin sensitivity [54,55]. In the present study, however, the serum levels of total FFAs were not correlated with serum glucose levels and were similar in AHF patients with T2D compared with those without this comorbidity. This is most likely due to the severe HF pathophysiology, which disrupts the associations between FFAs and glucose metabolism in our AHF patients.

There are several limitations to the present study: Due to the design, we could not examine causality for the relationship of FFAs with clinical and laboratory parameters. Since the nutritional state of our patients was unknown, we could not examine the impact of fasting/feeding on FFA levels and their associations with clinical and laboratory parameters. Considering the fact that almost 95% of our AHF patients belonged to NYHA class IV, our results do not reflect associations of FFAs with clinical and laboratory parameters in less severe AHF patients.

5. Conclusions

We conclude that individual and total serum FFAs are only slightly associated with established clinical and laboratory indicators of HF severity in patients with severe AHF

(NYHA class IV). Therefore, measurements of individual or total FFAs would not improve the estimation of the disease severity or risk in NYHA class IV AHF patients.

Supplementary Materials: The following supporting information can be downloaded at: https://www.mdpi.com/article/10.3390/biomedicines11123197/s1. Scheme S1: study flow chart; Table S1: chronic medication of AHF patients prior to index AHF hospitalization; Table S2: serum levels of FFAs in various groups of AHF patients; Table S3: differences in FFA levels between AHF patients who were alive and those who died during index AHF hospitalization or within 3 or 12 months after index AHF hospitalization.

Author Contributions: Conceptualization, S.F. and V.D.; Data curation, H.H. and G.P.; Formal analysis, G.P. and A.B.; Funding acquisition, S.F.; Investigation, I.K., H.H., M.L. and W.S.; Methodology, H.H., M.L. and W.S.; Project administration, S.F. and V.D.; Resources, I.K., M.T., W.S., S.F. and V.D.; Supervision, M.T., A.B., W.S., S.F. and V.D.; Validation, I.K.; Visualization, G.P.; Writing—original draft, S.F.; Writing—review and editing, I.K., H.H., M.L., M.T., G.P., A.B., W.S., S.F. and V.D. All authors have read and agreed to the published version of the manuscript.

Funding: This research was funded by the Medical University of Graz.

Institutional Review Board Statement: This study was conducted in accordance with the Declaration of Helsinki and approved by the Ethics Committee of the University Hospital Centre Sisters of Charity (EP 2258/18-10; 9 February 2018), Zagreb, Croatia, and the Medical University of Graz (33-258 ex 20/21; 16 February 2021) Graz, Austria.

Informed Consent Statement: Informed consent was obtained from all subjects involved in the study.

Data Availability Statement: Data are available within the article and Supplementary Materials.

Acknowledgments: We thank Celina Klampfer for her expert technical assistance.

Conflicts of Interest: The authors declare no conflict of interest.

References

1. Roger, V.L.; Weston, S.A.; Redfield, M.M.; Hellermann-Homan, J.P.; Killian, J.; Yawn, B.P.; Jacobsen, S.J. Trends in heart failure incidence and survival in a community-based population. *JAMA* **2004**, *292*, 344–350. [CrossRef]
2. Dickstein, K.; Cohen-Solal, A.; Filippatos, G.; McMurray, J.J.; Ponikowski, P.; Poole-Wilson, P.A.; Stromberg, A.; van Veldhuisen, D.J.; Atar, D.; Hoes, A.W.; et al. ESC Guidelines for the diagnosis and treatment of acute and chronic heart failure 2008: The Task Force for the Diagnosis and Treatment of Acute and Chronic Heart Failure 2008 of the European Society of Cardiology. Developed in collaboration with the Heart Failure Association of the ESC (HFA) and endorsed by the European Society of Intensive Care Medicine (ESICM). *Eur. Heart J.* **2008**, *29*, 2388–2442. [CrossRef] [PubMed]
3. McMurray, J.J.; Adamopoulos, S.; Anker, S.D.; Auricchio, A.; Bohm, M.; Dickstein, K.; Falk, V.; Filippatos, G.; Fonseca, C.; Gomez-Sanchez, M.A.; et al. ESC Guidelines for the diagnosis and treatment of acute and chronic heart failure 2012: The Task Force for the Diagnosis and Treatment of Acute and Chronic Heart Failure 2012 of the European Society of Cardiology. Developed in collaboration with the Heart Failure Association (HFA) of the ESC. *Eur. Heart J.* **2012**, *33*, 1787–1847. [CrossRef] [PubMed]
4. Ponikowski, P.; Voors, A.A.; Anker, S.D.; Bueno, H.; Cleland, J.G.F.; Coats, A.J.S.; Falk, V.; Gonzalez-Juanatey, J.R.; Harjola, V.P.; Jankowska, E.A.; et al. 2016 ESC Guidelines for the Diagnosis and Treatment of Acute and Chronic Heart Failure. *Rev. Esp. Cardiol.* **2016**, *69*, 1167. [CrossRef] [PubMed]
5. Packer, M. Pathophysiology of chronic heart failure. *Lancet* **1992**, *340*, 88–92. [CrossRef]
6. Mentz, R.J.; O'Connor, C.M. Pathophysiology and clinical evaluation of acute heart failure. *Nat. Rev. Cardiol.* **2016**, *13*, 28–35. [CrossRef]
7. Tang, W.H.; Mullens, W. Cardiorenal syndrome in decompensated heart failure. *Heart* **2010**, *96*, 255–260. [CrossRef]
8. Gnanaraj, J.F.; von Haehling, S.; Anker, S.D.; Raj, D.S.; Radhakrishnan, J. The relevance of congestion in the cardio-renal syndrome. *Kidney Int.* **2013**, *83*, 384–391. [CrossRef]
9. Mamic, P.; Chaikijurajai, T.; Tang, W.H.W. Gut microbiome—A potential mediator of pathogenesis in heart failure and its comorbidities: State-of-the-art review. *J. Mol. Cell. Cardiol.* **2021**, *152*, 105–117. [CrossRef]
10. Pasini, E.; Aquilani, R.; Testa, C.; Baiardi, P.; Angioletti, S.; Boschi, F.; Verri, M.; Dioguardi, F. Pathogenic Gut Flora in Patients With Chronic Heart Failure. *JACC Heart Fail.* **2016**, *4*, 220–227. [CrossRef]
11. Ambrosy, A.P.; Pang, P.S.; Khan, S.; Konstam, M.A.; Fonarow, G.C.; Traver, B.; Maggioni, A.P.; Cook, T.; Swedberg, K.; Burnett, J.C., Jr.; et al. Clinical course and predictive value of congestion during hospitalization in patients admitted for worsening signs and symptoms of heart failure with reduced ejection fraction: Findings from the EVEREST trial. *Eur. Heart J.* **2013**, *34*, 835–843. [CrossRef] [PubMed]

12. Niebauer, J.; Volk, H.D.; Kemp, M.; Dominguez, M.; Schumann, R.R.; Rauchhaus, M.; Poole-Wilson, P.A.; Coats, A.J.; Anker, S.D. Endotoxin and immune activation in chronic heart failure: A prospective cohort study. *Lancet* **1999**, *353*, 1838–1842. [CrossRef] [PubMed]
13. Doehner, W.; Frenneaux, M.; Anker, S.D. Metabolic impairment in heart failure: The myocardial and systemic perspective. *J. Am. Coll. Cardiol.* **2014**, *64*, 1388–1400. [CrossRef]
14. Szabo, T.; Postrach, E.; Mahler, A.; Kung, T.; Turhan, G.; von Haehling, S.; Anker, S.D.; Boschmann, M.; Doehner, W. Increased catabolic activity in adipose tissue of patients with chronic heart failure. *Eur. J. Heart Fail.* **2013**, *15*, 1131–1137. [CrossRef]
15. Sylvers-Davie, K.L.; Davies, B.S.J. Regulation of lipoprotein metabolism by ANGPTL3, ANGPTL4, and ANGPTL8. *Am. J. Physiol. Endocrinol. Metab.* **2021**, *321*, E493–E508. [CrossRef] [PubMed]
16. Gambert, S.; Vergely, C.; Filomenko, R.; Moreau, D.; Bettaieb, A.; Opie, L.H.; Rochette, L. Adverse effects of free fatty acid associated with increased oxidative stress in postischemic isolated rat hearts. *Mol. Cell. Biochem.* **2006**, *283*, 147–152. [CrossRef] [PubMed]
17. Steinberg, H.O.; Paradisi, G.; Hook, G.; Crowder, K.; Cronin, J.; Baron, A.D. Free fatty acid elevation impairs insulin-mediated vasodilation and nitric oxide production. *Diabetes* **2000**, *49*, 1231–1238. [CrossRef]
18. Opie, L.H.; Knuuti, J. The adrenergic-fatty acid load in heart failure. *J. Am. Coll. Cardiol.* **2009**, *54*, 1637–1646. [CrossRef]
19. Wende, A.R.; Brahma, M.K.; McGinnis, G.R.; Young, M.E. Metabolic Origins of Heart Failure. *JACC Basic Transl. Sci.* **2017**, *2*, 297–310. [CrossRef]
20. Karwi, Q.G.; Uddin, G.M.; Ho, K.L.; Lopaschuk, G.D. Loss of Metabolic Flexibility in the Failing Heart. *Front. Cardiovasc. Med.* **2018**, *5*, 68. [CrossRef]
21. Bertero, E.; Maack, C. Metabolic remodelling in heart failure. *Nat. Rev. Cardiol.* **2018**, *15*, 457–470. [CrossRef]
22. Lee, L.; Campbell, R.; Scheuermann-Freestone, M.; Taylor, R.; Gunaruwan, P.; Williams, L.; Ashrafian, H.; Horowitz, J.; Fraser, A.G.; Clarke, K.; et al. Metabolic modulation with perhexiline in chronic heart failure: A randomized, controlled trial of short-term use of a novel treatment. *Circulation* **2005**, *112*, 3280–3288. [CrossRef] [PubMed]
23. Zhang, L.; Lu, Y.; Jiang, H.; Zhang, L.; Sun, A.; Zou, Y.; Ge, J. Additional use of trimetazidine in patients with chronic heart failure: A meta-analysis. *J. Am. Coll. Cardiol.* **2012**, *59*, 913–922. [CrossRef] [PubMed]
24. Lopaschuk, G.D. Metabolic Modulators in Heart Disease: Past, Present, and Future. *Can. J. Cardiol.* **2017**, *33*, 838–849. [CrossRef] [PubMed]
25. Djousse, L.; Benkeser, D.; Arnold, A.; Kizer, J.R.; Zieman, S.J.; Lemaitre, R.N.; Tracy, R.P.; Gottdiener, J.S.; Mozaffarian, D.; Siscovick, D.S.; et al. Plasma free fatty acids and risk of heart failure: The Cardiovascular Health Study. *Circ. Heart Fail.* **2013**, *6*, 964–969. [CrossRef] [PubMed]
26. Degoricija, V.; Trbusic, M.; Potocnjak, I.; Radulovic, B.; Pregartner, G.; Berghold, A.; Scharnagl, H.; Stojakovic, T.; Tiran, B.; Frank, S. Serum concentrations of free fatty acids are associated with 3-month mortality in acute heart failure patients. *Clin. Chem. Lab. Med.* **2019**, *57*, 1799–1804. [CrossRef] [PubMed]
27. Yu, Y.; Jin, C.; Zhao, C.; Zhu, S.; Meng, S.; Ma, H.; Wang, J.; Xiang, M. Serum Free Fatty Acids Independently Predict Adverse Outcomes in Acute Heart Failure Patients. *Front. Cardiovasc. Med.* **2021**, *8*, 761537. [CrossRef] [PubMed]
28. Ouchi, S.; Miyazaki, T.; Shimada, K.; Sugita, Y.; Shimizu, M.; Murata, A.; Kato, T.; Aikawa, T.; Suda, S.; Shiozawa, T.; et al. Low Docosahexaenoic Acid, Dihomo-Gamma-Linolenic Acid, and Arachidonic Acid Levels Associated with Long-Term Mortality in Patients with Acute Decompensated Heart Failure in Different Nutritional Statuses. *Nutrients* **2017**, *9*, 956. [CrossRef]
29. Matsuo, N.; Miyoshi, T.; Takaishi, A.; Kishinoue, T.; Yasuhara, K.; Tanimoto, M.; Nakano, Y.; Onishi, N.; Ueeda, M.; Ito, H. High Plasma Docosahexaenoic Acid Associated to Better Prognoses of Patients with Acute Decompensated Heart Failure with Preserved Ejection Fraction. *Nutrients* **2021**, *13*, 371. [CrossRef]
30. Nagai, T.; Honda, Y.; Sugano, Y.; Nishimura, K.; Nakai, M.; Honda, S.; Iwakami, N.; Okada, A.; Asaumi, Y.; Aiba, T.; et al. Circulating Omega-6, But Not Omega-3 Polyunsaturated Fatty Acids, Are Associated with Clinical Outcomes in Patients with Acute Decompensated Heart Failure. *PLoS ONE* **2016**, *11*, e0165841. [CrossRef]
31. Ouchi, S.; Miyazaki, T.; Shimada, K.; Sugita, Y.; Shimizu, M.; Murata, A.; Kato, T.; Aikawa, T.; Suda, S.; Shiozawa, T.; et al. Decreased circulating dihomo-gamma-linolenic acid levels are associated with total mortality in patients with acute cardiovascular disease and acute decompensated heart failure. *Lipids Health Dis.* **2017**, *16*, 150. [CrossRef] [PubMed]
32. Hunter, W.G.; Kelly, J.P.; McGarrah, R.W., 3rd; Kraus, W.E.; Shah, S.H. Metabolic Dysfunction in Heart Failure: Diagnostic, Prognostic, and Pathophysiologic Insights from Metabolomic Profiling. *Curr. Heart Fail. Rep.* **2016**, *13*, 119–131. [CrossRef]
33. Lin, H.; Zhang, H.; Lin, Z.; Li, X.; Kong, X.; Sun, G. Review of nutritional screening and assessment tools and clinical outcomes in heart failure. *Heart Fail. Rev.* **2016**, *21*, 549–565. [CrossRef]
34. Denfeld, Q.E.; Winters-Stone, K.; Mudd, J.O.; Gelow, J.M.; Kurdi, S.; Lee, C.S. The prevalence of frailty in heart failure: A systematic review and meta-analysis. *Int. J. Cardiol.* **2017**, *236*, 283–289. [CrossRef]
35. Kalantar-Zadeh, K.; Block, G.; Horwich, T.; Fonarow, G.C. Reverse epidemiology of conventional cardiovascular risk factors in patients with chronic heart failure. *J. Am. Coll. Cardiol.* **2004**, *43*, 1439–1444. [CrossRef] [PubMed]
36. Voors, A.A.; Ouwerkerk, W.; Zannad, F.; van Veldhuisen, D.J.; Samani, N.J.; Ponikowski, P.; Ng, L.L.; Metra, M.; Ter Maaten, J.M.; Lang, C.C.; et al. Development and validation of multivariable models to predict mortality and hospitalization in patients with heart failure. *Eur. J. Heart Fail.* **2017**, *19*, 627–634. [CrossRef]

37. Lin, Y.; Pang, L.; Huang, S.; Shen, J.; Wu, W.; Tang, F.; Su, W.; Zhu, X.; Sun, J.; Quan, R.; et al. The prevalence and survival of pulmonary hypertension due to left heart failure: A retrospective analysis of a multicenter prospective cohort study. *Front. Cardiovasc. Med.* **2022**, *9*, 908215. [CrossRef]
38. Poudel-Tandukar, K.; Nanri, A.; Matsushita, Y.; Sasaki, S.; Ohta, M.; Sato, M.; Mizoue, T. Dietary intakes of alpha-linolenic and linoleic acids are inversely associated with serum C-reactive protein levels among Japanese men. *Nutr. Res.* **2009**, *29*, 363–370. [CrossRef]
39. Calder, P.C. Polyunsaturated fatty acids and inflammation. *Prostaglandins Leukot. Essent. Fat. Acids* **2006**, *75*, 197–202. [CrossRef]
40. Sacks, F.M.; Campos, H. Polyunsaturated fatty acids, inflammation, and cardiovascular disease: Time to widen our view of the mechanisms. *J. Clin. Endocrinol. Metab.* **2006**, *91*, 398–400. [CrossRef] [PubMed]
41. Takic, M.; Pokimica, B.; Petrovic-Oggiano, G.; Popovic, T. Effects of Dietary alpha-Linolenic Acid Treatment and the Efficiency of Its Conversion to Eicosapentaenoic and Docosahexaenoic Acids in Obesity and Related Diseases. *Molecules* **2022**, *27*, 4471. [CrossRef] [PubMed]
42. Djousse, L.; Khawaja, O.; Bartz, T.M.; Biggs, M.L.; Ix, J.H.; Zieman, S.J.; Kizer, J.R.; Tracy, R.P.; Siscovick, D.S.; Mukamal, K.J. Plasma fatty acid-binding protein 4, nonesterified fatty acids, and incident diabetes in older adults. *Diabetes Care* **2012**, *35*, 1701–1707. [CrossRef] [PubMed]
43. Carlsson, M.; Wessman, Y.; Almgren, P.; Groop, L. High levels of nonesterified fatty acids are associated with increased familial risk of cardiovascular disease. *Arter. Thromb. Vasc. Biol.* **2000**, *20*, 1588–1594. [CrossRef]
44. Fagot-Campagna, A.; Balkau, B.; Simon, D.; Warnet, J.M.; Claude, J.R.; Ducimetiere, P.; Eschwege, E. High free fatty acid concentration: An independent risk factor for hypertension in the Paris Prospective Study. *Int. J. Epidemiol.* **1998**, *27*, 808–813. [CrossRef] [PubMed]
45. Khawaja, O.; Bartz, T.M.; Ix, J.H.; Heckbert, S.R.; Kizer, J.R.; Zieman, S.J.; Mukamal, K.J.; Tracy, R.P.; Siscovick, D.S.; Djousse, L. Plasma free fatty acids and risk of atrial fibrillation (from the Cardiovascular Health Study). *Am. J. Cardiol.* **2012**, *110*, 212–216. [CrossRef]
46. Trico, D.; Mengozzi, A.; Nesti, L.; Hatunic, M.; Gabriel Sanchez, R.; Konrad, T.; Lalic, K.; Lalic, N.M.; Mari, A.; Natali, A.; et al. Circulating palmitoleic acid is an independent determinant of insulin sensitivity, beta cell function and glucose tolerance in non-diabetic individuals: A longitudinal analysis. *Diabetologia* **2020**, *63*, 206–218. [CrossRef]
47. Shramko, V.S.; Polonskaya, Y.V.; Kashtanova, E.V.; Stakhneva, E.M.; Ragino, Y.I. The Short Overview on the Relevance of Fatty Acids for Human Cardiovascular Disorders. *Biomolecules* **2020**, *10*, 1127. [CrossRef] [PubMed]
48. Lass, A.; Zimmermann, R.; Oberer, M.; Zechner, R. Lipolysis—A highly regulated multi-enzyme complex mediates the catabolism of cellular fat stores. *Prog. Lipid Res.* **2011**, *50*, 14–27. [CrossRef]
49. Henderson, G.C. Plasma Free Fatty Acid Concentration as a Modifiable Risk Factor for Metabolic Disease. *Nutrients* **2021**, *13*, 2590. [CrossRef]
50. Perry, R.J.; Samuel, V.T.; Petersen, K.F.; Shulman, G.I. The role of hepatic lipids in hepatic insulin resistance and type 2 diabetes. *Nature* **2014**, *510*, 84–91. [CrossRef]
51. Samuel, V.T.; Shulman, G.I. Nonalcoholic Fatty Liver Disease as a Nexus of Metabolic and Hepatic Diseases. *Cell Metab.* **2018**, *27*, 22–41. [CrossRef] [PubMed]
52. Krssak, M.; Falk Petersen, K.; Dresner, A.; DiPietro, L.; Vogel, S.M.; Rothman, D.L.; Roden, M.; Shulman, G.I. Intramyocellular lipid concentrations are correlated with insulin sensitivity in humans: A 1H NMR spectroscopy study. *Diabetologia* **1999**, *42*, 113–116. [CrossRef] [PubMed]
53. Korenblat, K.M.; Fabbrini, E.; Mohammed, B.S.; Klein, S. Liver, muscle, and adipose tissue insulin action is directly related to intrahepatic triglyceride content in obese subjects. *Gastroenterology* **2008**, *134*, 1369–1375. [CrossRef] [PubMed]
54. Schoiswohl, G.; Stefanovic-Racic, M.; Menke, M.N.; Wills, R.C.; Surlow, B.A.; Basantani, M.K.; Sitnick, M.T.; Cai, L.; Yazbeck, C.F.; Stolz, D.B.; et al. Impact of Reduced ATGL-Mediated Adipocyte Lipolysis on Obesity-Associated Insulin Resistance and Inflammation in Male Mice. *Endocrinology* **2015**, *156*, 3610–3624. [CrossRef]
55. Wu, J.W.; Wang, S.P.; Casavant, S.; Moreau, A.; Yang, G.S.; Mitchell, G.A. Fasting energy homeostasis in mice with adipose deficiency of desnutrin/adipose triglyceride lipase. *Endocrinology* **2012**, *153*, 2198–2207. [CrossRef]

biomedicines

MDPI

Article

Three-Dimensional Combined Atrioventricular Coupling Index—A Novel Prognostic Marker in Dilated Cardiomyopathy

Aura Vîjîiac [1,*], Alina Ioana Scărlătescu [2], Ioana Gabriela Petre [1,2], Cristian Vîjîiac [3] and Radu Gabriel Vătăşescu [1,2]

[1] Cardiology Department, Carol Davila University of Medicine and Pharmacy, 050474 Bucharest, Romania; i_comanescu@yahoo.com (I.G.P.); radu_vatasescu@yahoo.com (R.G.V.)
[2] Emergency Clinical Hospital Bucharest, 014461 Bucharest, Romania; alina.scarlatescu@gmail.com
[3] Emergency County Hospital Ploieşti, 100097 Ploieşti, Romania; cristivijiiac@yahoo.com
[*] Correspondence: aura.apostolescu@yahoo.com; Tel.: +40-752298189

Abstract: Atrioventricular coupling has recently emerged as an outcome predictor. Our aim was to assess, through three-dimensional (3D) echocardiography, the role of the left atrioventricular coupling index (LACI), right atrioventricular coupling index (RACI) and a novel combined atrioventricular coupling index (CACI) in a cohort of patients with dilated cardiomyopathy (DCM). One hundred twenty-one consecutive patients with DCM underwent comprehensive 3D echocardiographic acquisitions. LACI was defined as the ratio between left atrial and left ventricular 3D end-diastolic volumes. RACI was defined as the ratio between right atrial and right ventricular 3D end-diastolic volumes. CACI was defined as the sum of LACI and RACI. Patients were prospectively followed for death, heart transplant, nonfatal cardiac arrest and hospitalization for heart failure. Fifty-five patients reached the endpoint. All three coupling indices were significantly more impaired in patients with events, with CACI showing the highest area under the curve (AUC = 0.66, $p = 0.003$). All three indices were independent outcome predictors when tested in multivariable Cox regression (HR = 2.62, $p = 0.01$ for LACI; HR = 2.58, $p = 0.004$ for RACI; HR = 2.37, $p = 0.01$ for CACI), but only CACI showed an incremental prognostic power over traditional risk factors such as age, left ventricular strain, right ventricular strain and mitral regurgitation severity (likelihood ratio χ^2 test = 28.2, $p = 0.03$). CACI assessed through 3D echocardiography, reflecting both left and right atrioventricular coupling, is an independent predictor of adverse events in DCM, yielding an incremental prognostic power over traditional risk factors.

Keywords: dilated cardiomyopathy; atrioventricular coupling; three-dimensional echocardiography; combined atrioventricular coupling index

1. Introduction

Dilated cardiomyopathy (DCM) is a heterogeneous disease that still causes substantial morbidity and mortality worldwide [1]. Since it was mainly considered a disease of the left ventricle (LV), most of the research focused on the evaluation of LV function, with the LV ejection fraction (LVEF) having a well-established prognostic role in DCM [2,3]. However, ventricular and atrial dysfunction are closely intertwined. Left atrial (LA) volume and strain are not only markers of LV diastolic dysfunction but also independent outcome predictors in heart failure (HF) [4,5]. Moreover, recent data have shown that both right ventricular (RV) and right atrial (RA) dysfunction have an independent prognostic role in left-sided HF [6–8].

The physiological interplay between the atrium and the ventricle suggests that the assessment of atrioventricular coupling could better reveal myocardial dysfunction and improve the outcome prediction [9]. A novel cardiac magnetic resonance (CMR)-derived left atrioventricular coupling index (LACI), defined as the ratio between LA end-diastolic volume (EDV) and LV EDV, proved to be an independent predictor of adverse events in patients without cardiovascular disease [9] and in patients with myocardial infarction [10]. Although three-dimensional (3D) LV and LA volumes showed a good correlation with CMR measurements [11], LACI has not been assessed so far using 3D echocardiography, and its utility in DCM is unknown. There is no data regarding the 3D right atrioventricular coupling index (RACI), defined as the ratio between RA EDV and RV EDV [12]. Therefore, the aim of our study was to assess, through 3D echocardiography, the prognostic role of LACI, RACI and a novel combined atrioventricular coupling index (CACI) in patients with DCM.

2. Materials and Methods

2.1. Study Population

The study population consisted of consecutive adult patients with DCM referred to our echocardiography laboratory between January 2019 and December 2021. Inclusion criteria were as follows: a dilated LV, according to cutoffs proposed in the current chamber quantification guidelines [13], with LVEF < 40%, in the absence of significant coronary artery disease or severe valvular heart disease [14]. All patients provided written informed consent prior to enrollment. Exclusion criteria included poor acoustic window, inability to hold breath, persistent atrial fibrillation, cor pulmonale and life expectancy < 1 year. The study protocol was approved by the ethics committee of our hospital.

2.2. Echocardiography

Comprehensive two-dimensional (2D) and 3D echocardiographic acquisitions were performed using a Vivid E95 (GE Vingmed, Horten, Norway) ultrasound machine equipped with a 2.5 MHz 2D matrix array transducer and a 4V probe. Images were obtained with the patient in the left-lateral decubitus position, according to current recommendations [15], and they were subsequently analyzed offline using dedicated software (EchoPAC BT 13).

LVEF and 2D LV volumes were measured using Simpson's biplane disk summation rule from apical views [13,15]. LA and RA 2D volumes were obtained from the apical four-chamber view using the area-length method, providing the maximal volume (LA V_{max} and RA V_{max}) at ventricular end-systole, the minimal volume (LA V_{min} and RA V_{min}) at ventricular end-diastole, and the preA volume (LA V_{preA} and RA V_{preA}) at the peak of the P wave on ECG [13]. The mitral E/E′ ratio was measured using the average tissue Doppler diastolic velocity of the mitral annulus at septal and lateral annular sites. Mitral regurgitation (MR) severity was graded as mild, moderate or severe based on qualitative and semiquantitative criteria proposed in current guidelines [16]. We used the apical RV-focused view [15,17] to measure the tricuspid annular plane systolic excursion (TAPSE) and pulsed tissue Doppler systolic velocity of the tricuspid annulus (S wave). RA pressure was estimated using the inferior vena cava diameter and collapsibility from the subcostal view. Pulmonary artery systolic pressure (PASP) was estimated as the sum of RA pressure and the tricuspid regurgitation systolic gradient [17].

For strain analysis, we used 2D strain software (EchoPAC—Q Analysis package) using high frame rate acquisitions (50–70 frames per second). For the assessment of LV global longitudinal strain (GLS-LV), apical four-, two- and three-chamber views were acquired, and the software automatically traced the endocardial border, which was manually readjusted when needed. The average peak systolic strain of all LV segments was reported as GLS-LV [18]. RV strain was calculated as the average of the peak systolic strain of the RV free wall segments (RVFW-LS).

For 3D analysis, three experienced sonographers obtained six-beat full-volume 3D data sets with electrocardiographic gating during breath holding. For the left chambers, images were obtained from the apical four-chamber view, whereas for the right chambers, images were obtained from the apical RV-focused view. Datasets were analyzed offline using commercially available software: 4D Auto LVQ (EchoPAC v204, GE Vingmed, Horten, Norway) for LV analysis, 4D Auto RVQ (EchoPAC v204, GE Vingmed, Horten, Norway) for RV analysis and 4D Auto LAQ (EchoPAC v204, GE Vingmed, Horten, Norway) for

LA and RA analysis. The software thus provided the biventricular EDV, ESV, EF, and the biatrial V_{max}, V_{min} and V_{preA} at the same time in the cardiac cycle as the corresponding 2D volumes.

Based on the 3D atrial and ventricular volumes (Figure 1), we measured three atrioventricular coupling indices as follows: LACI, defined as the ratio between LA V_{min} and LV EDV; RACI, defined as the ratio between RA V_{min} and RV EDV; and CACI, defined as the sum between LACI and RACI. All the coupling indices were expressed as percentages, and a higher coupling index indicates a greater degree of atrioventricular decoupling.

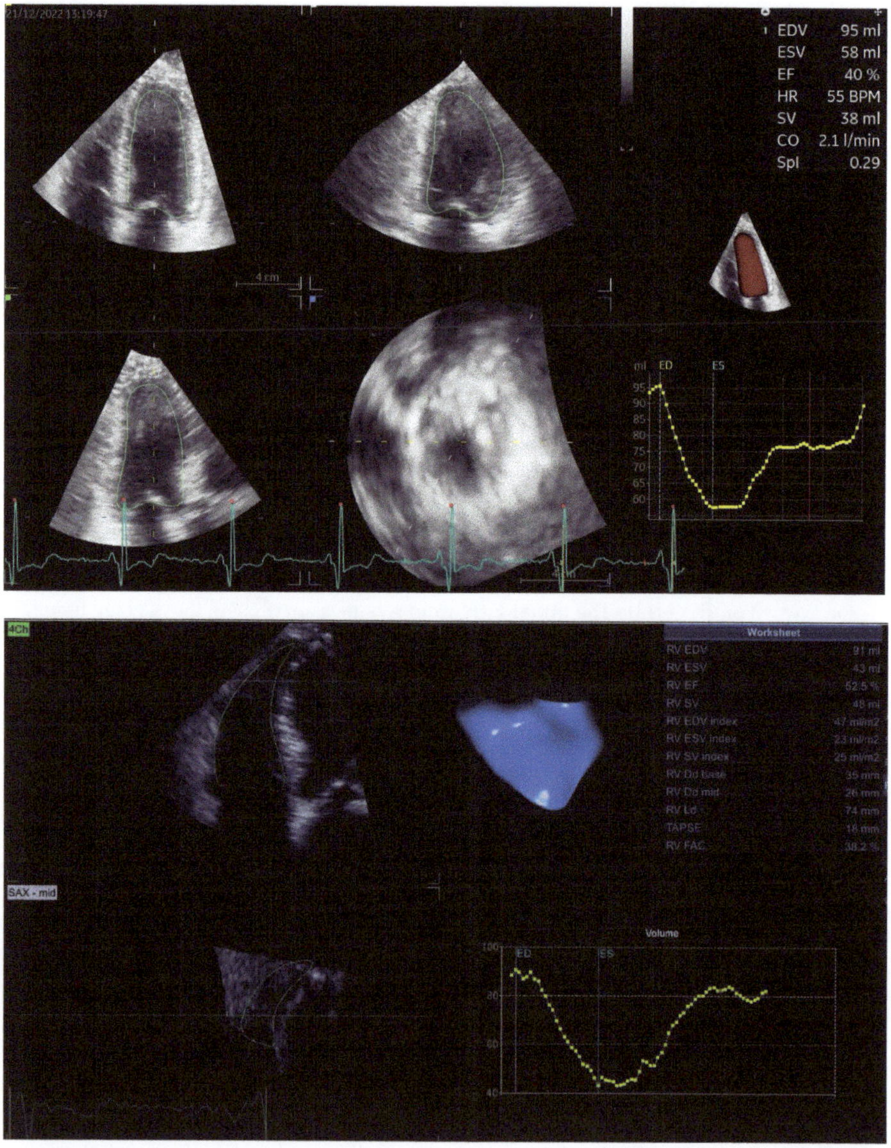

Figure 1. *Cont.*

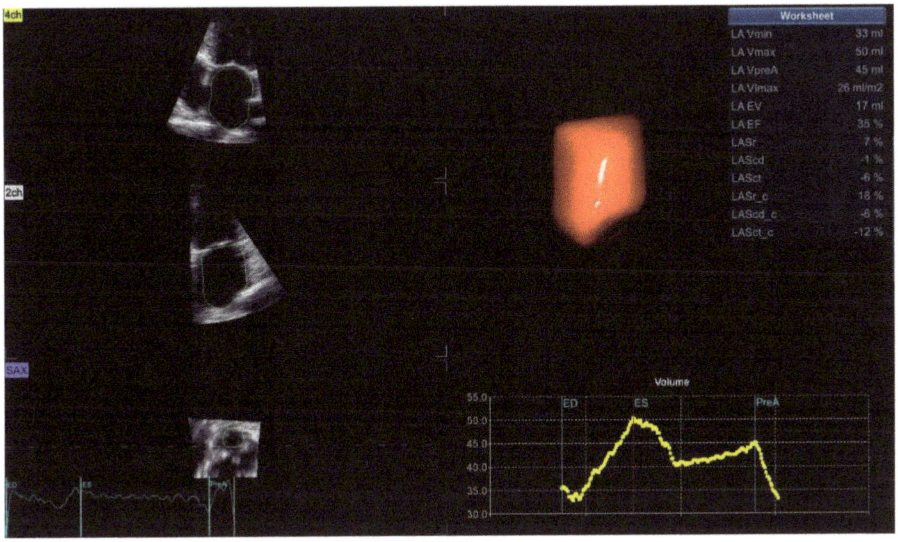

Figure 1. 3D assessment using dedicated software for analysis of LV volumes and EF (**upper panel**), RV volumes and EF (**middle panel**) and atrial volumes (**lower panel**), upon which measurements of LACI, RACI and CACI are based. Abbreviations are in the text.

3D acquisitions required an additional scanning time of 6 ± 3 min, while post-processing and offline analysis of biatrial and biventricular volumes required an additional 10 ± 4 min for each subject.

2.3. Follow-Up

Patients were followed up prospectively for the occurrence of any major adverse clinical event (MACE). The endpoint of this study was a composite of all-cause death, heart transplant, nonfatal cardiac arrest or readmission for heart failure exacerbation. For patients without MACE, we used the date of the last contact in survival analysis. Follow-up was conducted for a median of 19 ± 11 months.

2.4. Statistical Analysis

Statistical analysis was performed using SPSS version 20.0 statistical software package and GraphPad Prism version 10.0.0 software. The Kolmogorov–Smirnov test was used to check for normal distribution. Continuous data were presented as mean ± standard deviation or as median and interquartile range, depending on the distribution. Categorical data were displayed as numbers and percentages. Comparison between continuous variables was conducted with Student's *t*-test or Mann–Whitney U test, as dictated by distribution, while categorical variables were compared with Fisher exact test or χ^2 test, as appropriate.

Time-dependent receiver operating characteristic (ROC) curves and the respective area under the curve (AUC) were used to compare the ability of different parameters to predict the adverse outcome. Optimal cutoff values were chosen using the Youden index. Kaplan–Meier survival curves were compared using log-rank statistics.

Atrioventricular coupling indices were tested in univariable and multivariable Cox proportional hazards regression. The multivariable model was constructed using variables with clinical relevance and/or statistical significance in univariable regression. To examine the incremental prognostic value of LACI, RACI and CACI over well-established predictors in DCM, we constructed nested models and compared them with the likelihood ratio χ^2 test. A two-tailed p-value < 0.05 was considered statistically significant.

We assessed the intra- and interobserver reproducibility of 3D measurements using intraclass coefficients (ICC) on a two-way mixed-effects model. Interobserver reproducibility was evaluated by having 10 datasets analyzed by two different researchers. Intraobserver reproducibility was tested using repeated measurements of 10 datasets two weeks apart, performed by the same researcher.

3. Results

After the exclusion of patients with persistent atrial fibrillation (15 patients), cor pulmonale (10 patients), severe clinical status with inability to hold breath (18 patients), poor acoustic window (7 patients) and life expectancy < 1 year (2 patients), 121 patients with DCM in sinus rhythm formed the final study population. The baseline clinical characteristics are summarized in Table 1. Most patients were male (74%), and most were in NYHA class II (59%), with a mean age of 59 ± 14 years. Seventy-eight patients (65%) had been diagnosed with DCM less than one year prior to enrollment. The etiology of DCM in the study group was heterogenous; there were 19 patients (16%) with familial cardiomyopathy, 21 patients (17%) with alcohol-induced cardiomyopathy, 13 patients (11%) with post-myocarditis DCM, 10 patients (8%) with tachycardiomyopathy, 7 patients (6%) with dyssynchrnopathy, 4 patients (3%) with chemotherapy-induced cardiomyopathy, 2 patients (2%) with LV noncompaction and 45 patients (37%) with idiopathic DCM.

Table 1. Baseline clinical characteristics.

Variables	All Patients (n = 121)	MACE (n = 55)	No MACE (n = 66)	*p*
Age (years)	59 ± 14	59 ± 15	59 ± 14	0.92
Male, n (%)	89 (74%)	40 (73%)	49 (74%)	0.85
Comorbidities, n (%)				
Diabetes	29 (24%)	15 (27%)	14 (21%)	0.44
Hypertension	81 (6%)	33 (60%)	48 (73%)	0.14
Smoking	44 (36%)	20 (36%)	24 (36%)	1.00
Systolic BP (mm Hg)	125 ± 19	122 ± 19	128 ± 18	**0.047**
Diastolic BP (mm Hg)	80 (65–80)	70 (60–80)	80 (70–85)	**0.001**
Heart rate (bpm)	81 ± 16	82 ± 16	79 ± 15	0.35
NYHA class, n (%)				
II	71 (59%)	22 (40%)	49 (74%)	**<0.001**
III	43 (35%)	27 (49%)	16 (24%)	
IV	7 (6%)	6 (11%)	1 (2%)	
Medication, n (%)				
ACE-I/ARBs/ARN-I	115 (95%)	52 (95%)	63 (95%)	0.82
β blockers	117 (97%)	51 (93%)	66 (100%)	**0.04**
MRA	108 (89%)	51 (93%)	57 (86%)	0.26
SGLT2-I	17 (14%)	7 (13%)	10 (15%)	0.70
Loop diuretics	79 (65%)	44 (80%)	35 (53%)	**0.002**
NT pro-BNP (pg/mL)	480 (163–1525)	690 (211–1815)	253 (105–505)	**0.008**

Units of measurement are in parentheses. Abbreviations are in the text. Bolded *p* values are statistically significant.

Fifty-five patients (46%) experienced at least one MACE during follow-up; there were 26 deaths (22%), one heart transplant (1%), 5 nonfatal cardiac arrests (4%) and 23 readmissions for heart failure exacerbation (19%). Patients with events had a higher prevalence of NYHA class III and IV at enrollment ($p < 0.001$), a higher prevalence of diuretic use ($p = 0.002$) and higher brain natriuretic peptides (BNP) levels ($p = 0.008$). Except for diuretics, there were no differences regarding classes of HF drugs between patients with and without events (Table 1).

Table 2 presents 2D echocardiographic characteristics. There were no differences in LV systolic function between patients with and without events. However, patients with MACE had more severe LV diastolic dysfunction ($p < 0.001$ for mitral E/E′ ratio) and more impaired RV systolic function ($p < 0.001$ for TAPSE, S wave and RVFW-LS). All 2D LA and RA volumes were significantly larger in patients with events.

Table 2. 2D echocardiographic characteristics.

Variables	All Patients (n = 121)	MACE (n = 55)	No MACE (n = 66)	*p*
2D LVEDV index (mL/m^2)	125 ± 45	132 ± 49	118 ± 40	0.10
2D LVESV index (mL/m^2)	95 ± 40	102 ± 44	89 ± 36	0.07
2D LVEF (%)	25 ± 7	24 ± 7	26 ± 7	0.08
Mitral E/E′ ratio	16 ± 7	18 ± 8	13 ± 5	**<0.001**
MR severity, n (%)				0.06
Mild	87 (72%)	34 (62%)	53 (80%)	
Moderate	26 (21%)	17 (31%)	9 (14%)	
Severe	8 (7%)	4 (7%)	4 (6%)	
GLS-LV (%)	−6.8 ± 2.8	−6.3 ± 3.1	−7.2 ± 2.5	0.09
2D LA V_{max} index (mL/m^2)	52 ± 25	61 ± 25	45 ± 22	**<0.001**
2D LA V_{min} index (mL/m^2)	35 ± 20	42 ± 20	30 ± 18	**<0.001**
2D LA V_{preA} index (mL/m^2)	43 ± 21	50 ± 21	37 ± 20	**<0.001**
RV basal diameter (mm)	39 ± 8	41 ± 8	38 ± 7	0.08
TAPSE (mm)	17 (15–20)	16 (12–18)	19 (17–23)	**<0.001**
S wave (cm/s)	11 ± 3	9 ± 2	12 ± 2	**<0.001**
2D RA V_{max} index (mL/m^2)	29 (20–40)	34 (21–46)	25 (18–37)	**0.02**
2D RA V_{min} index (mL/m^2)	17 (11–27)	21 (12–31)	15 (10–23)	**0.02**
2D RA V_{preA} index (mL/m^2)	23 (16–34)	28 (17–38)	19 (15–31)	**0.009**
PASP (mm Hg)	41 ± 17	45 ± 18	38 ± 16	**0.04**
RVFW-LS (%)	−13.9 ± 8.1	−11.0 ± 8.4	−16.4 ± 7.1	**<0.001**

Units of measurement are in parentheses. Abbreviations are in the text. Bolded *p* values are statistically significant.

Table 3 presents 3D echocardiographic characteristics. There were excellent correlations between 2D and 3D LV volumes (r = 0.98, $p < 0.001$ for EDV; r = 0.99, $p < 0.001$ for ESV) and EF (r = 0.89, $p < 0.001$). All 2D LA volumes were positively correlated with the corresponding 3D volumes (r = 0.93, $p < 0.001$ for V_{min} and V_{max}; r = 0.94, $p < 0.001$ for V_{preA}). There were also excellent correlations between all 2D RA volumes and their corresponding 3D volumes (r = 0.96, $p < 0.001$ for V_{max}; r = 0.97, $p < 0.001$ for V_{preA} and V_{min}). All 3D LA and RA volumes were significantly larger in patients with MACE. While there were no differences in 3D LVEF between patients with and without events ($p = 0.22$), RVEF was significantly more impaired in patients with adverse outcomes (35 ± 8% versus 47 ± 7%, $p < 0.001$). All atrioventricular coupling indices were significantly larger in patients with MACE ($p = 0.009$ for LACI; $p = 0.005$ for RACI; $p = 0.003$ for CACI), reflecting a greater degree of decoupling.

Table 3. 3D echocardiographic characteristics.

Variables	All Patients (n = 121)	MACE (n = 55)	No MACE (n = 66)	p
3D LVEDV index (mL/m^2)	133 ± 48	142 ± 52	124 ± 43	**0.046**
3D LVESV index (mL/m^2)	100 ± 43	109 ± 46	93 ± 38	**0.047**
3D LVEF (%)	26 ± 7	25 ± 7	26 ± 7	0.22
3D LA V_{max} index (mL/m^2)	54 (39–66)	60 (51–72)	47 (31–59)	**<0.001**
3D LA V_{min} index (mL/m^2)	38 ± 20	44 ± 20	33 ± 19	**0.002**
3D LA V_{preA} index (mL/m^2)	44 (33–56)	50 (41–61)	36 (24–51)	**<0.001**
3D RVEDV index (mL/m^2)	83 ± 32	85 ± 35	81 ± 29	0.44
3D RVESV index (mL/m^2)	48 ± 20	55 ± 23	43 ± 16	**0.001**
3D RVEF (%)	42 ± 9	35 ± 8	47 ± 7	**<0.001**
3D RA V_{max} index (mL/m^2)	35 ± 20	41 ± 24	30 ± 14	**0.007**
3D RA V_{min} index (mL/m^2)	18 (12–29)	24 (15–34)	16 (11–25)	**0.003**
3D RA V_{preA} index (mL/m^2)	25 (17–36)	31 (20–42)	21 (14–32)	**0.004**
LACI (%)	26 (17–40)	29 (22–41)	22 (16–36)	**0.009**
RACI (%)	23 (16–40)	28 (19–45)	19 (15–30)	**0.005**
CACI (%)	51 (36–80)	59 (44–97)	42 (34–61)	**0.003**

Units of measurement are in parentheses. Abbreviations are in the text. Bolded p values are statistically significant.

Good intra- and interobserver reproducibility were found for LACI (ICC = 0.94 [95% CI, 0.78–0.98] and ICC = 0.95 [95% CI, 0.81–0.99], respectively), RACI (ICC = 0.93 [95% CI, 0.75–0.98] and ICC = 0.85 [95% CI, 0.51–0.96], respectively) and CACI (ICC = 0.95 [95% CI, 0.83–0.99] and ICC = 0.91 [95% CI, 0.66–0.98], respectively).

In unadjusted Cox regression (Table 4), most of the 2D and 3D LA and RA volumes were significant predictors of MACE. All three atrioventricular coupling indices were significant predictors in univariable analysis ($p = 0.005$ for LACI; $p = 0.03$ for RACI; $p = 0.006$ for CACI). ROC analysis was used to compare the prognostic power of atrioventricular coupling indices (Table 5) and to find optimal cutoffs for event prediction based on the Youden index. CACI showed the best AUC (AUC = 0.66, $p = 0.003$), closely followed by RACI (AUC = 0.65, $p = 0.005$) and LACI (AUC = 0.64, $p = 0.009$). A CACI higher than 44% had a 78% sensitivity and a 52% specificity for MACE prediction. Kaplan–Meier curves showed a higher risk of events in patients with higher LACI, RACI and CACI (log-rank $p = 0.001$ for all) (Figure 2).

Table 4. Unadjusted Cox regression for MACE.

Variables	HR (95% CI)	p
2D LVEDV	1.00 (1.00–1.01)	0.09
2D LVESV	1.00 (1.00–1.01)	**0.04**
2D LVEF	0.95 (0.92–0.99)	**0.01**
GLS-LV	1.15 (1.04–1.27)	**0.009**
RVFW-LS	1.08 (1.05–1.12)	**<0.001**
2D LA V_{max}	1.01 (1.00–1.01)	**0.001**
2D LA V_{min}	1.01 (1.00–1.02)	**0.001**
2D LA V_{preA}	1.01 (1.00–1.01)	**0.001**
2D RA V_{max}	1.01 (1.00–1.01)	**0.004**

Table 4. *Cont.*

Variables	HR (95% CI)	*p*
2D RA V_{min}	1.01 (1.00–1.02)	**0.003**
2D RA V_{preA}	1.01 (1.00–1.01)	**0.002**
3D LVEDV	1.00 (1.00–1.01)	**0.04**
3D LVESV	1.00 (1.00–1.01)	**0.03**
3D LVEF	0.97 (0.93–1.00)	0.08
3D RVEDV	1.00 (1.00–1.01)	0.30
3D RVESV	1.01 (1.01–1.02)	**<0.001**
3D RVEF	0.87 (0.84–0.90)	**<0.001**
3D LA V_{max}	1.01 (1.00–1.01)	**<0.001**
3D LA V_{min}	1.01 (1.00–1.02)	**0.001**
3D LA V_{preA}	1.01 (1.00–1.02)	**<0.001**
3D RA V_{max}	1.01 (1.00–1.01)	**0.003**
3D RA V_{min}	1.01 (1.00–1.02)	**0.002**
3D RA V_{preA}	1.01 (1.00–1.02)	**0.001**
LACI	1.02 (1.01–1.04)	**0.005**
LACI > 20%	3.21 (1.57–6.59)	**0.001**
RACI	1.01 (1.00–1.02)	**0.03**
RACI > 21%	2.63 (1.47–4.68)	**0.001**
CACI	1.01 (1.00–1.02)	**0.005**
CACI > 44%	2.91 (1.53–5.55)	**0.001**

HR—hazard ratio; CI—confidence interval. The rest of the abbreviations are in the text. Bolded *p* values are statistically significant.

Table 5. ROC analysis for MACE prediction.

Variables	AUC (95% CI)	*p*	Cut-Off	Sensitivity	Specificity
LACI	0.64 (0.54–0.74)	0.009	20%	84%	44%
RACI	0.65 (0.55–0.75)	0.005	21%	71%	58%
CACI	0.66 (0.56–0.76)	0.003	44%	78%	52%

AUC—area under the curve; CI—confidence interval. The rest of the abbreviations are in the text.

All 3D atrial volumes and atrioventricular coupling indices were analyzed in multivariable Cox regression (Table 6). They were not tested together in the same model to avoid collinearity issues. The constructed model included well-established clinical and echocardiographic predictors in DCM (age, GLS-LV, MR severity and RVFW-LS) and, alternatively, one atrial volume or one atrioventricular coupling index at a time. We included GLS-LV and not LVEF in the model to avoid collinearity issues. None of the 3D LA volumes were independent predictors of MACE, while 3D RA V_{min} and RA V_{preA} remained independent outcome predictors. LACI, RACI and CACI were all independently associated with adverse events when tested as a categorical variable, but only CACI kept its prognostic power when tested as a continuous variable (Table 6).

The likelihood ratio χ^2 test demonstrated an incremental value of CACI (χ^2 = 28.2, p = 0.03) to predict adverse outcomes on top of the multivariable model, including age, GLS-LV, MR severity and RVFW-LS (Figure 3). LACI and RACI yielded no incremental value (p = 0.07 and p = 0.08, respectively).

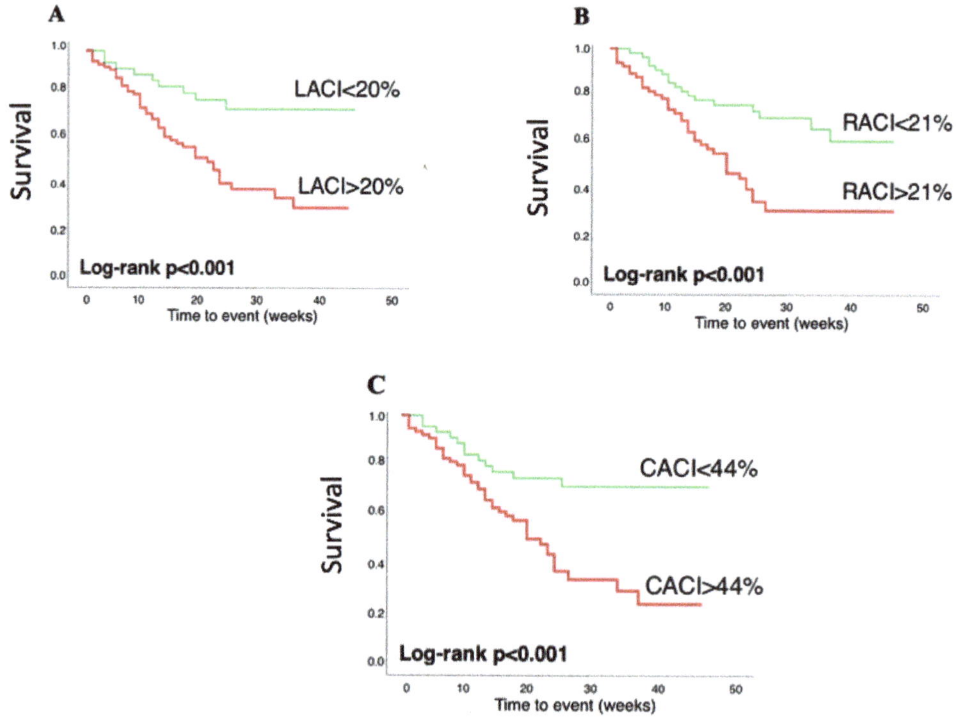

Figure 2. Kaplan–Meier survival curves stratified using left atrioventricular coupling index (**A**), right atrioventricular coupling index (**B**) and combined atrioventricular coupling index (**C**).

Table 6. Adjusted * Cox regression for MACE.

Variables	HR (95% CI)	*p*
3D LA V_{max}	1.01 (1.00–1.01)	0.06
3D LA V_{min}	1.01 (1.00–1.01)	0.14
3D LA V_{preA}	1.01 (1.00–1.01)	0.08
3D RA V_{max}	1.01 (1.00–1.01)	0.06
3D RA V_{min}	1.01 (1.00–1.02)	**0.046**
3D RA V_{preA}	1.01 (1.00–1.02)	**0.03**
CACI > 44% (yes/no)	2.37 (1.20–4.70)	**0.01**
CACI (per unit increase)	1.01 (1.00–1.02)	**0.03**
LACI > 20% (yes/no)	2.62 (1.22–5.60)	**0.01**
LACI (per unit increase)	1.02 (1.00–1.04)	0.07
RACI > 21% (yes/no)	2.58 (1.36–4.90)	**0.004**
RACI (per unit increase)	1.01 (1.00–1.03)	0.09

* Adjusted for age, GLS-LV, MR severity and RVFW-LS. HR—hazard ratio; CI—confidence interval. The rest of the abbreviations are in the text. Bolded *p* values are statistically significant.

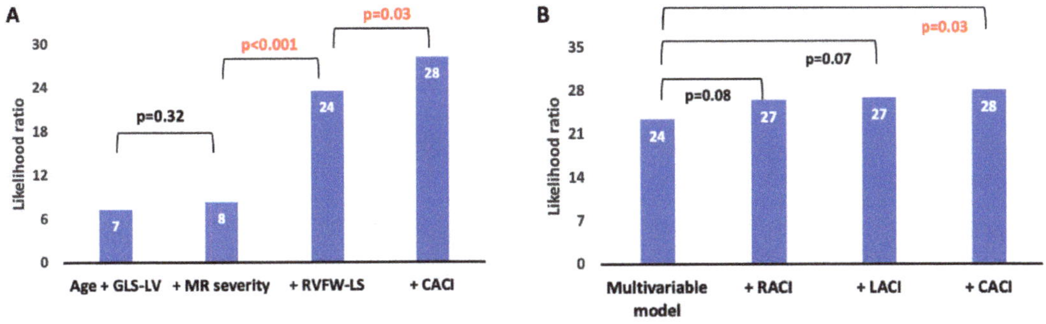

Figure 3. Bar charts showing the incremental prognostic value of atrioventricular coupling indices over traditional prognostic factors presented as a likelihood ratio χ^2 test. (**A**) The addition of RVFW-LS and subsequently of CACI over nested models, including age, GLS-LV and MR severity, led to significant incremental prognostic power. (**B**) The addition of CACI, but neither LACI nor RACI, yielded an incremental prognostic value over the multivariable model, including age, GLS-LV, MR severity and RVFW-LS.

4. Discussion

In this study, we found that 3D left and right atrioventricular coupling indices, as well as a novel 3D combined atrioventricular coupling index, were independent predictors of MACE in a cohort of patients with DCM. CACI showed the best association with adverse outcomes, having an incremental predictive value over traditional risk factors.

The atrioventricular coupling index describes the hemodynamic relationship between the atrium and the ventricle in diastole [9]. The morphology and physiology of the LA reflect LV filling pressure and diastolic function [19,20]. While LA ESV is usually communicated in echo reports, since it is a well-known outcome predictor and marker of the chronicity of LV dysfunction [21,22], recent studies suggest that LA EDV is a better correlate of ventricular filling pressure and a better prognostic marker [4,23,24]. Moreover, a high LA EDV indicates an impaired atrial booster pump function. The change in atrial volume relative to that of the ventricle reflects the ventricular compliance, which in turn influences the atrial reservoir function, and LACI detects an earlier stage of atrial remodeling than atrial volumes alone [25]. Since it is based on the simultaneous measurement of LA and LV volume, LACI is supposed to integrate more accurately the atrial and ventricular performance [10], and it was proven to detect patients with heart failure and preserved LVEF with high diagnostic accuracy [26].

Based on these pathophysiological considerations, Pezel et al. investigated the role of CMR-derived LACI in a large cohort of patients free from cardiovascular disease at enrollment and found that this parameter was a strong predictor of incident heart failure [25] and major cardiovascular events [9]. CMR-derived LACI was also recently investigated in patients with cardiovascular disease, and it proved to be an independent predictor of adverse outcomes in patients with abnormal vasodilator stress CMR [27] and in patients following acute myocardial infarction, particularly in high-risk patients with LVEF <35% [10]. LACI was also assessed with cardiac CT, and it proved to be an independent predictor of cardiac death in a healthy population [28]. Meucci et al. recently found that LACI measured by 2D echocardiography was a strong predictor of atrial fibrillation in patients with hypertrophic cardiomyopathy [29]. However, 2D LA volumetric assessment is less accurate than 3D assessment because the atrium does not dilate uniformly; 3D echocardiography provides more precise measurements, free from geometric assumptions or atrial foreshortening [30]. Despite these advantages of 3D over 2D echocardiography, our study is the first assessment of atrioventricular coupling using 3D echocardiography. So far, the only other evaluation of RACI was undertaken using CMR in a cohort of pediatric patients with repaired tetralogy of Fallot, and it showed that CMR-derived RACI was a predictor of malignant arrhythmias [12].

Our study is the first evaluation of atrioventricular coupling in patients with DCM. The optimal LACI cutoff for event prediction was 20%, lower than the cutoffs found in the abovementioned studies (most of which were, however, based on CMR), which ranged from 25% to 40% [9,10,29]. The most likely explanation is the fact that DCM is a disease involving primarily the LV, leading to important ventricular dilation, often disproportionately when compared to the dilation of the LA. Therefore, LACI in DCM will fall within a lower range than in other cardiac diseases. More studies are needed to establish reference ranges for LACI and RACI across the spectrum of cardiac pathologies. So far, our study is the first evaluation of both LACI and RACI in the same cohort.

The LA dilation and functional impairment in DCM are adaptative changes in response to LV dysfunction, but they may be partly explained using intrinsic atrial cardiomyopathy. The same is true for the RV, which undergoes morpho-functional changes secondary to afterload increase but which can also be affected by the same myopathic process as the LV. These changes in the RV will, in turn, lead to an impairment of RA function. In our study, LVEDV and RVEDV did not differ significantly between patients with and without MACE; however, LA and RA end-diastolic volumes (2D and 3D) were significantly larger in patients with events, suggesting different atrial adaptation patterns in response to impaired ventricular function. However, atrial volumes did not remain independent predictors in multivariable regression, while atrioventricular coupling indices did. The novel CACI, which was first described and investigated in the current study, showed the highest incremental predictive value when added over traditional risk factors. Furthermore, it was the only coupling index that retained its prognostic power when tested both as a categorical and as a continuous variable. This index considers changes in all four heart chambers; this can partly explain its prognostic value in our study since DCM is a disease that alters the morphology and function of all heart chambers. However, this is the first evaluation of CACI, and its predictive accuracy must be validated in larger external cohorts.

4.1. Clinical Implications

Since atrioventricular coupling proved to have better predictive value than atrial and ventricular volumes taken separately, early detection of atrioventricular mismatch should improve risk stratification in DCM. For this purpose, the novel CACI is probably the best choice because it includes both left and right atrioventricular decoupling. Since it is a unitless parameter, it should be easily reproducible among different 3D vendors, but further studies are needed. While 3D echocardiography is not yet routinely performed for all DCM patients, it did become more available and utilized during the last decade, and an advantage of CACI is that its measurement is based on volumes that are routinely reported in a 3D study.

4.2. Study Limitations

While having the advantage of its prospective design, our study should be interpreted in the context of several limitations. It is a single-center experience with a small sample size and a relatively short follow-up period. Selection bias cannot be fully excluded since we did not include patients with atrial fibrillation to avoid stitch artifacts in 3D acquisitions. Moreover, there are no reference values in the general population for LACI, RACI and CACI, and the cutoffs derived from our ROC analysis are most likely not applicable to other cardiac diseases. Last but not least, the prognostic power of CACI was rather modest, and its potential impact on clinical decision-making remains to be determined.

5. Conclusions

Greater CACI measured with 3D echocardiography, indicative of left and right atrioventricular mismatch, was an independent predictor of major cardiovascular events in patients with DCM, showing an incremental prognostic power over traditional risk factors.

Author Contributions: Conceptualization, A.V.; methodology, A.V. and R.G.V.; formal analysis, C.V.; investigation, A.I.S. and I.G.P.; data curation, A.V., A.I.S. and I.G.P.; writing—original draft preparation, A.V. and C.V.; writing—review and editing, A.I.S. and R.G.V.; supervision, R.G.V. All authors have read and agreed to the published version of the manuscript.

Funding: This research was supported by CREDO Project—ID: 49182, financed by the National Authority of Scientific Research and Innovation, on behalf of the Romanian Ministry of European Funds—through the Sector Operational Program "Increasing of Economic Competitiveness", Priority Axis 2, Operation 2.2.1 (SOP IEC-A2-0.2.2.1-2013-1) co-financed by the European Regional Development Fund.

Institutional Review Board Statement: This study was conducted in accordance with the Declaration of Helsinki and approved by the Ethics Committee of Emergency Clinical Hospital Bucharest, approval number 7817/22.10.2018.

Informed Consent Statement: Informed consent was obtained from all subjects involved in the study.

Data Availability Statement: Data are available upon request.

Conflicts of Interest: The authors declare no conflicts of interest.

References

1. Maron, B.J.; Towbin, J.A.; Thiene, G.; Thiene, G.; Antzelevitch, C.; Corrado, D.; Arnett, D.; Moss, A.J.; Seidman, C.E.; Young, J.B. Contemporary definitions and classification of the cardiomyopathies: An American Heart Association Scientific Statement from the Council on Clinical Cardiology, Heart Failure and Transplantation Committee; Quality of Care and Outcomes Research and Function. *Circulation* **2006**, *113*, 1807–1816. [CrossRef] [PubMed]
2. Curtis, J.P.; Sokol, S.I.; Wang, Y.; Rathore, S.S.; Ko, D.T.; Jadbabaie, F.; Portnay, E.L.; Marshalko, S.J.; Radford, M.J.; Krumholz, H.M. The association of left ventricular ejection fraction, mortality, and cause of death in stable outpatients with heart failure. *J. Am. Coll. Cardiol.* **2003**, *42*, 736–742. [CrossRef] [PubMed]
3. McDonagh, T.A.; Metra, M.; Adamo, M.; Gardner, R.S.; Baumbach, A.; Bohm, M.; Burri, H.; Butler, J.; Celutkiene, J.; Chioncel, O.; et al. 2021 ESC Guidelines for the diagnosis and treatment of acute and chronic heart failure. *Eur. Heart J.* **2021**, *42*, 3599–3726. [CrossRef] [PubMed]
4. Prasad, S.B.; Guppy-Coles, K.; Stanton, T.; Armstrong, J.; Krishnaswamy, R.; Whalley, G.; Atherton, J.J.; Thomas, L. Relation of Left Atrial Volumes in Patients with Myocardial Infarction to Left Ventricular Filling Pressures and Outcomes. *Am. J. Cardiol.* **2019**, *124*, 325–333. [CrossRef]
5. Bisbal, F.; Baranchuk, A.; Braunwald, E.; Bayes de Luna, A.; Bayes-Genis, A. Atrial Failure as a Clinical Entity: JACC Review Topic of the Week. *J. Am. Coll. Cardiol.* **2020**, *75*, 222–232. [CrossRef]
6. Vîjîiac, A.; Onciul, S.; Guzu, C.; Verinceanu, V.; Bataila, V.; Deaconu, S.; Scarlatescu, A.; Zamfir, D.; Petre, I.; Onut, R.; et al. The prognostic value of right ventricular longitudinal strain and 3D ejection fraction in patients with dilated cardiomyopathy. *Int. J. Cardiovasc. Imaging* **2021**, *37*, 3233–3244. [CrossRef]
7. Vîjîiac, A.; Vătășescu, R.; Onciul, S.; Guzu, C.; Verinceanu, V.; Petre, I.; Deaconu, S.; Scarlatescu, A.; Zamfir, D.; Scafa-Udriste, A.; et al. Right atrial phasic function and outcome in patients with heart failure and reduced ejection fraction: Insights from speckle-tracking and three-dimensional echocardiography. *Kardiol. Pol.* **2022**, *80*, 322–331. [CrossRef] [PubMed]
8. Seo, J.; Jung, I.H.; Park, J.H.; Kim, G.S.; Lee, H.Y.; Byun, Y.S.; Kim, B.O.; Rhee, K.J. The prognostic value of 2D strain in assessment of the right ventricle in patients with dilated cardiomyopathy. *Eur. Heart J. Cardiovasc. Imaging* **2019**, *20*, 1043–1050. [CrossRef]
9. Pezel, T.; Venkatesh, B.A.; De Vasconcellos, H.D.; Kato, Y.; Shabani, M.; Xie, E.; Heckbert, S.R.; Post, W.S.; Shea, S.J.; Allen, N.B.; et al. Left Atrioventricular Coupling Index as a Prognostic Marker of Cardiovascular Events: The MESA Study. *Hypertension* **2021**, *78*, 661–671. [CrossRef]
10. Lange, T.; Backhaus, S.J.; Schulz, A.; Evertz, R.; Kowallick, J.T.; Bigalke, B.; Hasenfuss, G.; Thiele, H.; Stiermaier, T.; Eitel, I.; et al. Cardiovascular magnetic resonance-derived left atrioventricular coupling index and major adverse cardiac events in patients following acute myocardial infarction. *J. Cardiovasc. Magn. Reson.* **2023**, *25*, 24. [CrossRef]
11. Zhao, D.; Quill, G.M.; Gilbert, K.; Wang, V.Y.; Houle, H.C.; Legget, M.E.; Ruygrok, P.N.; Doughty, R.N.; Pedrosa, J.; D'hooge, J.; et al. Systematic Comparison of Left Ventricular Geometry between 3D-Echocardiography and Cardiac Magnetic Resonance Imaging. *Front. Cardiovasc. Med.* **2021**, *8*, 728205. [CrossRef] [PubMed]
12. Gunsaulus, M.; Bueno, A.; Bright, C.; Snyder, K.; Das, N.; Dobson, C.; DeBrunner, M.; Cristopher, A.; Hoskoppal, A.; Follansbee, C.; et al. The Use of Automated Atrial CMR Measures and a Novel Atrioventricular Coupling Index for Predicting Risk in Repaired Tetralogy of Fallot. *Child* **2023**, *10*, 400. [CrossRef] [PubMed]

13. Lang, R.M.; Badano, L.P.; Mor-Avi, V.; Afilalo, J.; Armstrong, A.; Ernande, L.; Flachskampf, F.A.; Foster, E.; Goldstein, S.A.; Kuznetsova, T.; et al. Recommendations for cardiac chamber quantification by echocardiography in adults: An update from the American society of echocardiography and the European association of cardiovascular imaging. *Eur. Heart J. Cardiovasc. Imaging* **2015**, *16*, 233–271. [CrossRef] [PubMed]
14. Pinto, Y.M.; Elliott, P.M.; Arbustini, E.; Adler, Y.; Anastasakis, A.; Bohm, M.; Duboc, D.; Gimeno, J.; deGroote, P.; Imazio, M.; et al. Proposal for a revised definition of dilated cardiomyopathy, hypokinetic non-dilated cardiomyopathy, and its implications for clinical practice: A position statement of the ESC working group on myocardial and pericardial diseases. *Eur. Heart J.* **2016**, *37*, 1850–1858. [CrossRef] [PubMed]
15. Mitchell, C.; Rahko, P.S.; Blauwet, L.A.; Canaday, B.; Finstuen, J.A.; Foster, M.C.; Horton, K.; Ogunyankin, K.O.; Palma, R.A.; Velasquez, E.J. Guidelines for Performing a Comprehensive Transthoracic Echocardiographic Examination in Adults: Recommendations from the American Society of Echocardiography. *J. Am. Soc. Echocardiogr.* **2019**, *32*, 1–64. [CrossRef] [PubMed]
16. Zoghbi, W.A.; Adams, D.; Bonow, R.O.; Enriquez-Sarano, M.; Foster, E.; Grayburn, P.A.; Hahn, R.T.; Han, Y.; Hung, J.; Lang, R.M.; et al. Recommendations for Noninvasive Evaluation of Native Valvular Regurgitation: A Report from the American Society of Echocardiography Developed in Collaboration with the Society for Cardiovascular Magnetic Resonance. *J. Am. Soc. Echocardiogr.* **2017**, *30*, 303–371. [CrossRef] [PubMed]
17. Rudski, L.G.; Lai, W.W.; Afilalo, J.; Hua, L.; Handschumacher, M.D.; Chandrasekaran, K.; Solomon, S.D.; Louie, E.K.; Schiller, N.B. Guidelines for the Echocardiographic Assessment of the Right Heart in Adults: A Report from the American Society of Echocardiography. Endorsed by the European Association of Echocardiography, a registered branch of the European Society of Cardiology, and the Canadian Society of Echocardiography. *J. Am. Soc. Echocardiogr.* **2010**, *23*, 685–713.
18. Voigt, J.U.; Pedrizzetti, G.; Lysyansky, P.; Marwick, T.H.; Houle, H.; Baumann, R.; Pedri, S.; Ito, Y.; Abe, Y.; Metz, S.; et al. Definitions for a common standard for 2D speckle tracking echocardiography: Consensus document of the EACVI/ASE/Industry Task Force to standardize deformation imaging. *Eur. Heart J. Cardiovasc. Imaging* **2015**, *16*, 1–11. [CrossRef]
19. Barbier, P.; Solomon, S.B.; Schiller, N.B.; Glantz, S.A. Left atrial relaxation and left ventricular systolic function determine left atrial reservoir function. *Circulation* **1999**, *100*, 427–436. [CrossRef]
20. Inoue, K.; Khan, F.H.; Remme, E.W.; Ohte, N.; Garcia-Izquierdo, E.; Chetrit, M.; Monivas-Palomero, V.; Mingo-Santos, S.; Andersen, O.S.; Gude, E.; et al. Determinants of left atrial reservoir and pump strain and use of atrial strain for evaluation of left ventricular filling pressure. *Eur. Heart J. Cardiovasc. Imaging* **2021**, *23*, 61–70. [CrossRef]
21. Hoit, B.D. Left atrial size and function: Role in prognosis. *J. Am. Coll. Cardiol.* **2014**, *63*, 493–505. [CrossRef] [PubMed]
22. Katsiki, N.; Mikhailidis, D.P.; Papanas, N. Left atrial volume: An independent predictor of cardiovascular outcomes. *Int. J. Cardiol.* **2018**, *265*, 234–235. [CrossRef] [PubMed]
23. Habibi, M.; Samiei, S.; Ambale Venkatesh, B.; Opdahl, A.; Helle-Valle, T.M.; Zareian, M.; Almeida, A.L.; Choi, E.Y.; Wu, C.; Alonso, A.; et al. Cardiac Magnetic Resonance-Measured Left Atrial Volume and Function and Incident Atrial Fibrillation: Results from MESA (Multi-Ethnic Study of Atherosclerosis). *Circ. Cardiovasc. Imaging* **2016**, *9*, e004299. [CrossRef] [PubMed]
24. Ben-Arzi, A.; Hazanov, E.; Ghanim, D.; Rozen, G.; Marai, I.; Grosman-Rimon, L.; Kachel, E.; Amir, O.; Carasso, S. Left atrial minimal volume: Association with diastolic dysfunction and heart failure in patients in sinus rhythm or atrial fibrillation with preserved ejection fraction. *BMC Med. Imaging* **2021**, *21*, 76. [CrossRef] [PubMed]
25. Pezel, T.; Ambale Venkatesh, B.; Kato, Y.; De Vasconcellos, H.D.; Heckbert, S.R.; Wu, C.O.; Post, W.S.; Bluemke, D.A.; Cohen-Solal, A.; Henry, P.; et al. Left Atrioventricular Coupling Index to Predict Incident Heart Failure: The Multi-Ethnic Study of Atherosclerosis. *Front. Cardiovasc. Med.* **2021**, *8*, 76. [CrossRef] [PubMed]
26. Backhaus, S.J.; Lange, T.; Schulz, A.; Evertz, R.; Frey, S.M.; Hasenfuss, G.; Schuster, A. Cardiovascular magnetic resonance rest and exercise-stress left atrioventricular coupling index to detect diastolic dysfunction. *Am. J. Physiol. Heart Circ. Physiol.* **2023**, *324*, H686–H695. [CrossRef]
27. Pezel, T.; Garot, P.; Toupin, S.; Sanguineti, F.; Hovasse, T.; Unterseeh, T.; Champagne, S.; Morisset, S.; Chitiboi, T.; Jacob, A.J.; et al. AI-Based Fully Automated Left Atrioventricular Coupling Index as a Prognostic Marker in Patients Undergoing Stress CMR. *JACC Cardiovasc. Imaging* **2023**, *16*, 1288–1302. [CrossRef]
28. Pezel, T.; Dillinger, J.-G.; Toupin, S.; Mirailles, R.; Logeart, D.; Cohen-Solal, A.; Unger, A.; Canuti, E.S.; Beauvais, F.; Lafont, A.; et al. Left atrioventricular coupling index assessed using cardiac CT as a prognostic marker of cardiovascular death. *Diagn. Interv. Imaging* **2023**, *104*, 594–604. [CrossRef]
29. Meucci, M.; Fortuni, F.; Galloo, X.; Bootsma, M.; Crea, F.; Bax, J.J.; Marsan, N.A.; Delgado, V. Left atrioventricular coupling index in hypertrophic cardiomyopathy and risk of new-onset atrial fibrillation. *Eur. Heart J. Cardiovasc. Imaging* **2022**, *363*, 87–93.
30. Carpenito, M.; Fanti, D.; Mega, S.; Benfari, G.; Bono, M.C.; Rossi, A.; Ribichini, F.L.; Grigioni, F. The Central Role of Left Atrium in Heart Failure. *Front. Cardiovasc. Med.* **2021**, *8*, 704762. [CrossRef]

biomedicines

MDPI

Article

Comparative Temporal Analysis of Morbidity and Early Mortality in Heart Transplantation with Extracorporeal Membrane Oxygenation Support: Exploring Trends over Time

Raquel López-Vilella [1,2,*], Manuel Pérez Guillén [3], Borja Guerrero Cervera [2], Ricardo Gimeno Costa [4], Iratxe Zarragoikoetxea Jauregui [5], Francisca Pérez Esteban [4], Paula Carmona [5], Tomás Heredia Cambra [3], Mónica Talavera Peregrina [4], Azucena Pajares Moncho [5], Carlos Domínguez-Massa [3], Víctor Donoso Trenado [1,2], Luis Martínez Dolz [2,6], Pilar Argente [5], Álvaro Castellanos [4], Juan Martínez León [3], Salvador Torregrosa Puerta [3] and Luis Almenar Bonet [1,2,6]

1 Heart Failure and Transplant Unit, Hospital Universitari i Politècnic La Fe, 46026 Valencia, Spain; vdonoso@outlook.com (V.D.T.); lualmenar@gmail.com (L.A.B.)
2 Cardiology Department, Hospital Universitari i Politècnic La Fe, 46026 Valencia, Spain; borja_vlc95@hotmail.com (B.G.C.); martinez_luidol@gva.es (L.M.D.)
3 Cardiovascular Surgery Department, Hospital Universitari i Politècnic La Fe, 46026 Valencia, Spain; perez_mgui@gva.es (M.P.G.); tomheca@hotmail.com (T.H.C.); dominguez.massa@gmail.com (C.D.-M.); juan.martinez-leon@uv.es (J.M.L.); torregrosa_sal@gva.es (S.T.P.)
4 Intensive Care Department, Hospital Universitari i Politècnic La Fe, 46026 Valencia, Spain; ricardogimeno55@hotmail.com (R.G.C.); perez_fraest@gva.es (F.P.E.); talavera_mon@gva.es (M.T.P.); castellanos_alv@gva.es (Á.C.)
5 Department of Anesthesiology and Critical Care, Hospital Universitari i Politècnic La Fe, 46026 Valencia, Spain; iratxezarragoikoetxea@hotmail.com (I.Z.J.); paulac_g@hotmail.com (P.C.); pajares.maz@gmail.com (A.P.M.); argente_marnav@gva.es (P.A.)
6 Centro de Investigación Biomédica en Red de Enfermedades Cardiovasculares (CIBERCV), Instituto de Salud Carlos III, 28029 Madrid, Spain
* Correspondence: lopez_raqvil@gva.es

Abstract: Background/Objectives: The direct bridge to urgent heart transplant (HT) with venoarterial extracorporeal membrane oxygenation (VA-ECMO) support has been associated with high morbidity and mortality. The objective of this study is to analyze the morbidity and mortality of patients transplanted with VA-ECMO and compare the presumed differences between various eras over a 17-year timeline. Methods: This is a prospective, observational study on consecutive patients stabilized with VA-ECMO and transplanted with VA-ECMO from July 2007 to December 2023 at a reference center (98 patients). Objective variables were mortality and morbidity from renal failure, venous thromboembolic disease (VTD), primary graft dysfunction (PGD), the need for tracheostomy, severe myopathy, reoperation, post-transplant ECMO, vascular complications, and sepsis/infection. Results: The percentage of patients who reached transplantation without the need for mechanical ventilation has increased over the periods studied. No significant differences were found between the study periods in 30-day mortality ($p = 0.822$), hospital discharge ($p = 0.972$), one-year mortality ($p = 0.706$), or five-year mortality ($p = 0.797$). Survival rates in these periods were 84%, 75%, 64%, and 61%, respectively. Comorbidities were very frequent, with an average of 3.33 comorbidities per patient. The most frequent were vascular complications (58%), the need for post-transplant ECMO (57%), and myopathy (55%). The development of myopathy and the need for post-transplant ECMO were higher in recent periods ($p = 0.004$ and $p = 0.0001$, respectively). Conclusions: VA-ECMO support as a bridge to HT allows hospital discharge for 3 out of 4 transplanted patients. This survival rate has not changed over the years. The comorbidities associated with this device are frequent and significant.

Keywords: urgent heart transplantation; venoarterial extracorporeal membrane oxygenation; morbidity; mortality; eras

1. Introduction

Cardiogenic shock (CS) has been, for decades, one of the greatest challenges in critical cardiology. This condition presents a very high risk of significant morbidity and mortality despite the most current therapeutic advances [1,2]. In this context, circulatory assistance with extracorporeal membrane oxygenation in venoarterial configuration [VA-ECMO] has undoubtedly been a crucial intervention to provide circulatory and oxygenation support in refractory CS, especially in INTERMACS 1–2 cases [1,3,4]. In cases of non-recovery of myocardial function, an urgent heart transplant (HT) is often performed in patients supported with ECMO [5]. However, the morbidity associated with ECMO assistance is not negligible and is exacerbated by the complex profile of the patients who require its use [6–8]. In high-volume centers for VA-ECMO implantation, complications can be minimized, and it is possible that over time and with the team's experience, the survival and complications of patients undergoing HT with ECMO have changed. The objective of this study is to analyze the early global morbidity, mortality and eras of patients undergoing HT assisted by VA-ECMO in a long-term time series (17 years). The secondary objective is to analyze mid- to long-term mortality by time periods in the same patients.

2. Materials and Methods

This is a prospective, observational, non-interventional study in which all patients included on the heart transplant waiting list from July 2007 to December 2023 at a reference center (n = 503) were consecutively recruited. Patients who ultimately underwent HT without ECMO (n = 348), those undergoing combined HT (n = 18), re-transplants (n = 10), and pediatric transplants (<16 years, n = 17) were excluded. Patients who, after ECMO implantation, left the waiting list and were not transplanted, either due to death or other reasons (n = 12), were also excluded. Finally, 98 consecutive patients transplanted with VA-ECMO were included in the analysis. Figure 1 shows the patient flow. All transplants performed were recorded with variables considered in the Spanish Cardiac Transplant Registry [9]. Additionally, variables related to mechanical assistance were analyzed: type, days of assistance, related complications, etc. Urgency 0 or Code 0 implies priority over all other candidates nationwide to receive the first suitable available heart donor in the system and applies to patients in CS requiring short-term circulatory/ventricular assistance. The analysis was divided into time periods: the first from 2007 (the first VA-ECMO implanted as a bridge to transplant) to 2010. This period was chosen because the literature shows that the learning curve period in ECMO-implanting teams is about 3 years [10,11]. The other periods were from 2011 to 2016 and from 2017 to 2023.

Surgical cannulation was performed in the Intensive Care Unit as per the center's protocol, avoiding the need to transfer the unstable patient in CS to the operating room. In most patients, femoral access is used, with an arterial cannula introduced into the common femoral artery and a multi-perforated venous cannula into the femoral vein. For limb perfusion, a pediatric arterial cannula is used and connected to the ECMO arterial line. Some patients with a reduced femoral artery caliber require the placement of a Dacron graft, through which an arterial cannula is introduced, enabling simultaneous systemic and limb perfusion. In the past, the limb perfusion cannula was connected to the arterial cannula via a three-way stopcock, but now a 3/8-3/8-1/4 connection is used from the ECMO arterial line to arterial and limb perfusion cannulas to avoid the resistance that occurred with the three-way stopcock and to reduce thrombotic complications and limb ischemia. The cannulas are inserted into the femoral vessels after creating a purse-string suture with polypropylene, which is then secured with tourniquets tied to the arterial cannulas to prevent movement. In contrast, the venous cannula is not fixed to allow for repositioning if needed (Figure 2). Transthoracic echocardiography is used to confirm the correct positioning of the venous cannula entering the right atrium. Additionally, the cannulas are inserted through cutaneous counter incisions to allow for wound closure and prevent infection until ECMO weaning is possible. The procedure is performed with systemic heparinization using sodium heparin at a dose of 1 mg/kg. After 24–48 h, if no bleeding complications arise, the continuous infusion of sodium heparin is initiated.

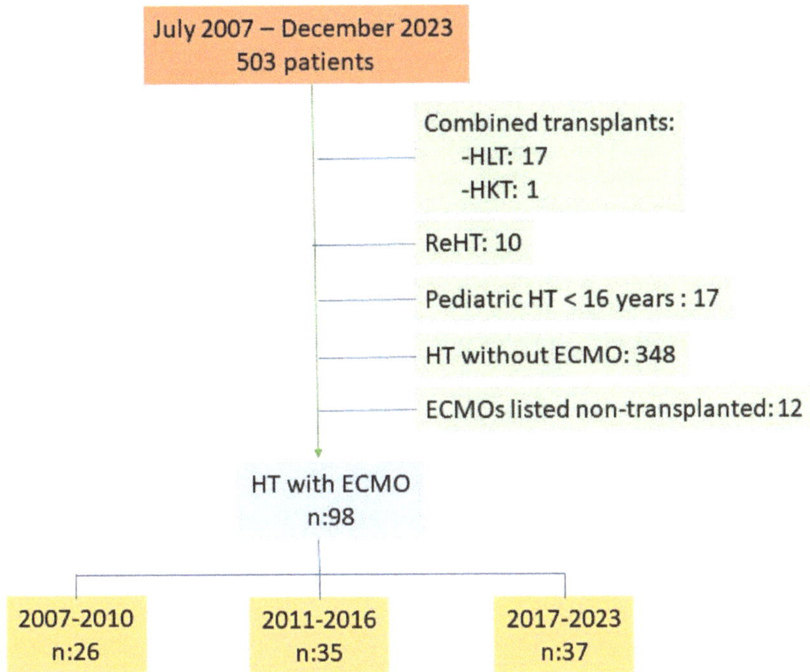

Figure 1. Study flowchart. Abbreviations: HLT: heart–lung transplantation; HKT: heart–kidney transplantation; and HT: heart transplantation.

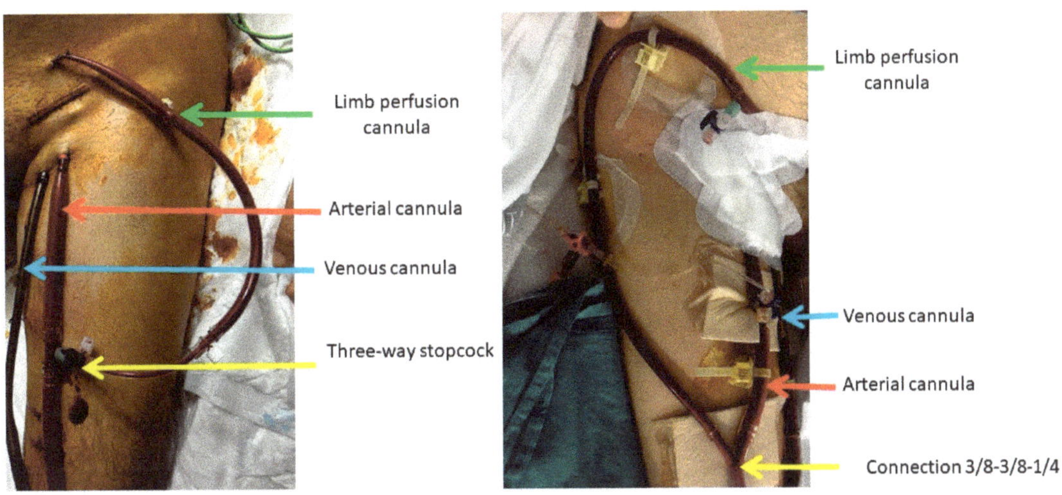

Figure 2. Venoarterial ECMO cannulation.

Early mortality was defined as that occurring within the first 30 days after HT. Hospital mortality was defined as death from any cause before discharge from HT admission. Mortality from any cause was also considered at one year and five years post-transplant. Primary graft dysfunction (PGD) was defined, according to the consensus published by ISHLT in 2014, as primary graft dysfunction excluding causes such as hyperacute rejection, pulmonary hypertension, or surgical complications, diagnosed within 24 h post-surgery [12]. Severe PGD, defined as requiring post-transplant mechanical assistance, was analyzed, which, in all cases, was performed using VA-ECMO. In the study center, in urgent HT with ECMO, it is maintained by the protocol for at least 24 h post-HT; however, PGD was only considered if the previous definition was met, including the verification of ventricular dysfunction with the inability to withdraw ECMO support in the first 24–48 h post-transplant. The definitions of the complications are detailed below. Infections were considered infectious processes with or without an identified microorganism that presented with symptoms, signs, or biomarkers of infection and required the initiation or expansion of antibiotic treatment for control. All cases of pulmonary embolism (PE) were confirmed by angio-CT $\pm$ pulmonary tree angiography, while all cases of deep vein thrombosis (DVT) were confirmed by vascular Doppler ultrasound. Post-transplant renal failure (RF) was defined as that requiring renal replacement therapy (RRT), including ultrafiltration and/or dialysis, at any time during transplant admission. Vascular complications included all complications related to the vascular access of the mechanical assistance(s) used by the patient. The study protocol was approved by the Ethics Committee of Hospital Universitari i Politècnic La Fe (Code ECMO-HF), Valencia.

Statistical Analysis

Qualitative variables are expressed as numbers and percentages, and quantitative variables as median and interquartile ranges (non-normal distribution, $p < 0.05$ in the Kolmogorov–Smirnov test). A comparison between quantitative variables was performed using Kruskal–Wallis ANOVA. For comparative analysis between qualitative variables, Pearson's Chi-square test was applied. Survival curves were calculated using the Kaplan–Meier method. A p-value of <0.05 was considered significant. Statistical analysis was performed using SPSS Statistics Version 27® software and Stata Statistics/Data Analysis 16.1, serial number 501606323439. Graphs were created using SPSS and PowerPoint. The database was designed with Excel and completed at patient discharge. PowerPoint and Excel are part of the Microsoft Office Professional Plus 2019 statistical package.

3. Results

3.1. Baseline Characteristics

The profile of the patients did not show significant variations over time (Table 1). The patients' age was similar across the three periods, around 55 years, and most were male, with ischemic heart disease being the predominant underlying etiology. However, from 2017 to 2023, the percentage of patients with ischemic heart disease was similar to those with dilated cardiomyopathy, familial, and other etiologies. The percentage of patients transplanted with mechanical ventilation (MV) was 64% and was lower in the most recent period (36% from 2017 to 2023). The duration of ECMO support was longer in the more recent periods, with a shorter duration (134 h) from 2007 to 2010. There were no differences in the main donor characteristics or surgical procedures, except for the use of the bicaval technique, which became increasingly common, reaching 89% in the last period.

3.2. Analysis of Overall Mortality and by Periods

Early mortality (day 30) did not significantly change over the years and was 19% from 2007 to 2010 and 14% from 2017 to 2023 ($p = 0.822$). No significant differences were found in mortality until hospital discharge (overall series: 25%), at one year (overall series: 36%), and five years (overall series: 39%). These results are shown in Table 2. Figure 3 shows survival over the study period for the three analyzed periods.

Table 1. Clinical characteristics of patients (overall and by eras).

	2007–2010 (n: 26)	2011–2016 (n: 35)	2017–2023 (n: 37)	*p*	Overall (n: 98)
Recipient					
Age (years) #	58 (11)	54 (21)	51 (14)	0.242	55 (15)
Male (n, %)	16 (62)	26 (74)	28 (76)	0.425	70 (71)
Underlying etiology (n, %)				0.474	
ischemic	13 (50)	18 (51)	13 (35)		44 (45)
Idiopathic + familial DCM	7 (27)	11 (31)	13 (35)		31 (32)
Other	6 (23)	6 (18)	11 (30)		23 (23)
Creatinine (mg/dL) #	0.9 (0.8)	0.7 (0.7)	0.7 (0.3)	0.124	0.8 (0.6)
AST (U/L) #	70 (53)	55 (36)	39 (39)	0.178	54 (45)
ALT (U/L) #	59 (94)	38 (44)	47 (83)	0.365	51 (69)
Bilirrubin (mg/dL) #	1.4 (1.5)	2.2 (1.9)	1.3 (1.5)	0.004	1.6 (1.6)
Pre-transplant infection (n, %)	8 (31)	13 (37)	7 (19)	0.254	28 (29)
I-D Diabetes (n, %)	0 (0)	3 (9)	2 (5)	0.445	5 (5)
MV (n, %)	26 (100)	25 (71)	12 (32)	0.001	63 (64)
Previous sternotomy (n, %)	2 (7)	5 (14)	6 (16)	0.724	13 (13)
ECMO duration (hours) #	134 (128)	204 (219)	192 (120)	0.004	192 (147)
Donor					
Donor age (years)	43 (24)	46 (16)	46 (15)	0.173	45 (17)
Donor cause of death (n, %)				0.345	
TBI	5 (19)	10 (29)	9 (24)		25 (24)
Stroke	20 (77)	23 (66)	22 (59)		65 (66)
Other	1 (4)	2 (5)	6 (17)		9(10)
Surgical Procedure					
CPB time (min) #	135 (53)	139 (42)	115 (39)	0.107	128 (43)
Ischemia time (min) #	200 (50)	192 (97)	189 (79)	0.444	192 (83)
Bicaval technique (n, %)	14 (54)	24 (69)	33 (89)	0.002	71 (72)

Median and interquartile range. Statistical test: Kruskal–Wallis ANOVA and Pearson's Chi-square test. Abbreviations: ALT: alanine aminotransferase; AST: aspartate aminotransferase; CPB: cardiopulmonary bypass; DCM: dilated cardiomyopathy; ECMO: extracorporeal membrane oxygenation; I-D: insulin-dependent; MV: mechanical ventilation; TBI: traumatic brain injury.

Table 2. Mortality analysis.

Variables	2007–2010 (n: 26)	2011–2016 (n: 35)	2017–2023 (n: 37)	*p*	Overall (n: 98)
Mortality at 30 days (n, %)	5 (19)	6 (17)	5 (14)	0.822	16 (16)
In-hospital mortality (n, %)	6 (23)	9 (26)	9 (24)	0.972	24 (25)
Mortality at one year (n, %)	9 (35)	13 (38)	12 (36)	0.706	34 (36)
Mortality at five years (n, %)	10 (39)	15 (43)	13 (35)	0.797	38 (39)

In each period, the mortality values are cumulative. Statistical test: Pearson's Chi-square test.

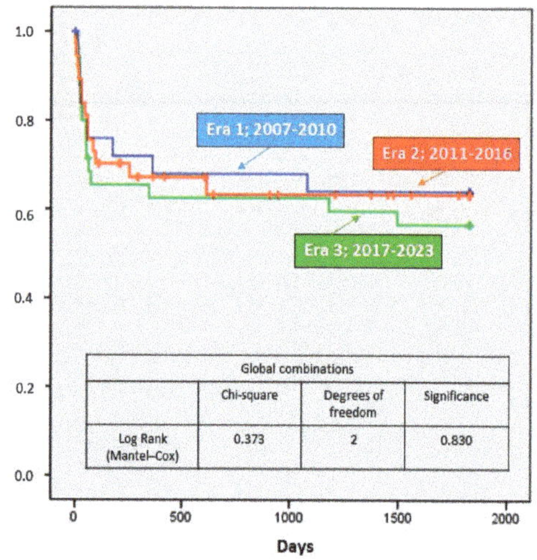

Figure 3. Survival at thirty days, one year, and five years.

3.3. *Analysis of Morbidity*

The overall prevalence of complications in patients with pre-transplant ECMO was generally very high, with an average frequency of 3.3 complications per patient. The percentage of patients without any of the analyzed complications was less than 10% (Figure 4). No differences were observed in the development of PE, DVT, PGD, vascular complications, or infections/sepsis (Table 3). However, in the periods from 2011 to 2016 and 2017 to 2023, there was a trend toward a lower prevalence of renal failure and a higher proportion of patients requiring tracheostomy and reoperation for bleeding and/or tamponade. In the periods from 2011 to 2016 and 2017 to 2023, there was a higher frequency of severe myopathy and the need for post-transplant mechanical support, both of which were statistically significant ($p = 0.004$ and $p = 0.0001$, respectively). The duration (hours) of pre-transplant ECMO correlated with the need for tracheostomy, with a trend toward other complications, such as the need for post-transplant ECMO, PGD, vascular complications, reoperation for bleeding, and sepsis (Figure 5).

Table 3. Morbidity analysis.

Variables	2007–2010 (n: 26)	2011–2016 (n: 35)	2017–2023 (n: 37)	p	Overall (n: 98)
Renal failure (n, %)	15 (58)	12 (34)	15 (41)	0.177	42 (43)
DVP ± EP (n, %)	2 (8)	0 (0)	4 (11)	0.058	6 (6)
PGD (n, %)	5 (19)	5 (14)	9 (24)	0.560	19 (19)
Tracheostomy (n, %)	4 (15)	11 (31)	13 (35)	0.208	28 (29)
Severe myopathy/polyneuropathy (n, %)	8 (31)	19 (54)	27 (73)	0.004	54 (55)
Reintervention for bleeding/tamponade (n, %)	6 (23)	17 (49)	18 (49)	0.077	41 (42)
Post-transplant ECMO (n, %)	5 (19)	25 (71)	26 (70)	0.001	56 (57)
Vascular complications * (n, %)	16 (62)	21 (60)	20 (54)	0.808	57 (58)
Sepsis/infection (n, %)	6 (23)	12 (34)	10 (27)	0.610	28 (29)

* Includes hemorrhages and compartment syndrome. Statistical test: Pearson's Chi-square test. Abbreviations: DVT: deep vein thrombosis; ECMO: extracorporeal membrane oxygenation; PE: pulmonary embolism; PGD: primary graft dysfunction.

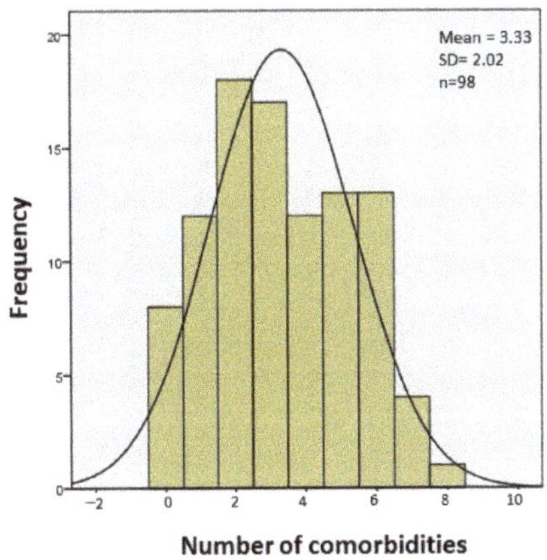

Figure 4. Overall prevalence of complications in patients pre-transplant (complications per patient). The histogram shows the percentage of patients presenting each number of complications.

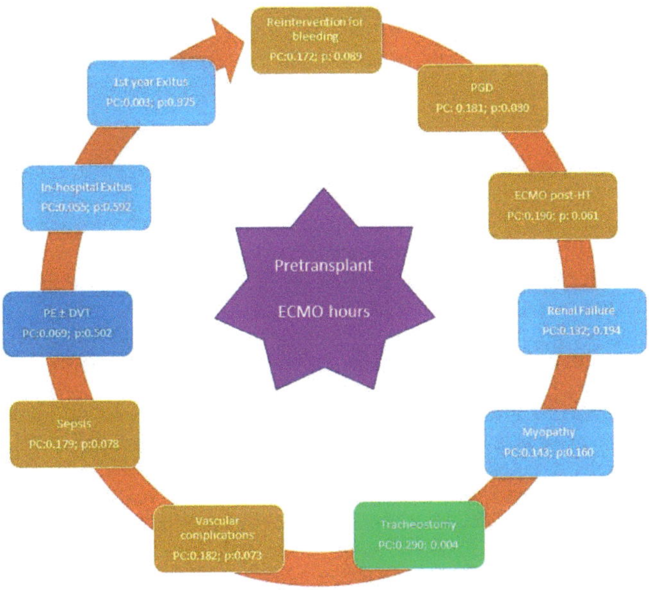

Figure 5. Association between complications and duration of pre-transplant ECMO support. Statistically significant associations are shown in green, trends in yellow, and associations without statistical significance in blue (Pearson correlation). Abbreviations: DVT: deep vein thrombosis; ECMO: extracorporeal membrane oxygenation; EP: pulmonary embolism; PC: Pearson correlation; PGD: primary graft dysfunction.

4. Discussion

CS represents the most extreme form of cardiac failure, where inadequate cardiac output compromises the perfusion of tissues and organs. Short-term mortality for patients with heart failure (HF) remains above 30% [13–15]. In this situation, in addition to inotropic drugs, ventricular and/or circulatory assist devices are required while determining the most appropriate therapeutic approach. In fact, in these patients, especially those at INTERMACS 1 [16], the direct implantation of long-term left ventricular assist devices is associated with a high mortality rate, around 60–70% in the first year. For this reason, in these profiles, it is recommended to implant short-term mechanical support until the patient is more stabilized, either as a bridge to heart transplantation or as a bridge to long-term ventricular assist devices [17,18]. For the most urgent cases that require rapid action, ECMO has marked a turning point by reducing mortality in these patients, particularly when circulatory support is needed while awaiting the appearance of a donor as a bridge to HT [19]. However, this device, in its venoarterial variant, is not without complications and morbidity. This study aimed to assess, over a prolonged series of 17 years, the survival of patients with VA-ECMO who undergo transplantation across various eras and the comorbidities associated with the use of this device. It has been observed that, over the years, the clinical characteristics of patients have not varied, with a hospital mortality rate of 25% and an average of 3.3 relevant comorbidities per patient.

The average clinical profile of patients in this series is a male around 55 years old. Other studies offer a slightly higher age range [20–22]. The majority of them reach transplantation without mechanical ventilation in the most recent period (32%). This fact reduces the risk of mortality [23,24]. In the Spanish ASIS-TC study, the average waiting time with short-term assistance until urgent CT was 7.6 days [21], which is a time similar to that of our series, which stood at 8 days, although it should be noted that 10% were excluded from the waiting list and were not transplanted. There were no differences regarding the main characteristics of the donor or the surgical procedure, except for the use of the bicaval technique. The bicaval technique in heart transplantation offers several advantages over the classical (biatrial) technique, such as the better anatomical alignment of the recipient's atria compared with those of the donor, the preservation of the anatomy of both atria, the reduced incidence of tricuspid regurgitation due to the preservation of the integrity of the annular anatomy, and improved sinus node function [25,26]. However, the choice of technique may depend on the surgeon's experience and the specific characteristics of the patient and donor.

In the analyzed series, early mortality did not significantly vary over the years, being 19% from 2007 to 2010 and 14% in the most recent period. This early mortality is lower than that observed in analyses conducted on urgent HT with ECMO. In the ASIS-TC study, in-hospital mortality was 33.3% in this patient group [21]. In a study by Rousse N et al., with fewer patients, in-hospital mortality in this group was 38.5% [27]. It is very likely that early mortality in transplantation with ECMO is significantly influenced by the selection of the candidate patient and the experience of the center. Medium- and long-term mortality (1 and 5 years) is also similar across periods. A 2020 study analyzed heart transplants in adults performed in the United States between 2005 and 2017 using the UNOS database; a survival analysis was conducted to compare patients bridged to transplantation with different modalities. Of the 24,905 adult transplants performed, unadjusted 1-year post-transplant survival was 68 $\pm$ 3% in ECMO, which is similar to the overall rate in this series (64%) [28]. Lui et al. conducted a recent study using the UNOS database of all adult patients requiring VA-ECMO support before HT between 2001 and 2018; with 118 ECMO-supported transplants, a significant decrease in 1-year survival was found [29]. Overall, mortality in our series was lower than that reported in other studies. In this regard, it should be noted that a recent study found higher mortality rates in centers that did not perform long-term transplantation/assistance (65.5% compared to 55.8% in centers that performed long-term transplantation/assistance) [30]. It should be noted that it is known that urgent heart transplants have a worse initial prognosis, while in the long term, patients who survive tend to have a better prognosis, as they are usually younger and more carefully selected patients. In the latest report from the Spanish Heart Transplant Registry, urgent HT increases the mortality of the procedure with a hazard ratio of 1.3 [31].

The overall prevalence of complications in patients with pre-transplant ECMO was generally high, with an average frequency of 3.3 complications per patient. There were no observed differences between eras in the development of PE, DVT, acute limb ischemia, femoral arteriovenous fistula, femoral stenosis, vascular complications, or infections/sepsis.

A recent study evaluated the frequency of vascular complications (arterial and venous) following ECMO removal using Doppler ultrasound on all patients, with a median support duration of 8 days; DVT was found in 41% and arterial complications in 14% (including 9 cases of acute limb ischemia, 1 femoral arteriovenous fistula, and 5 cases of late femoral stenosis) [32]. This series collectively analyzed DVT and vascular complications, finding a prevalence of 54% in the last era analyzed. Regarding post-transplant infections in patients undergoing urgent HT, it is estimated that infectious complications could affect slightly more than half of the ECMO-treated patients and those using short-term mechanical assist devices [33,34]. In this series, the prevalence of post-transplant infections in urgent ECMO cases was 29%, which is similar to that reported in a recent multicenter study, which found that nearly 35% of patients undergoing urgent CT with short-term assistance had a total of 102 infections, 26% of which involved ECMO [35]. Infections are estimated to complicate between 30% and 55% of ECMO treatments and impact survival [34,36]. Ventilator-associated pneumonia is the most frequent nosocomial infection in patients receiving veno-venous ECMO [36]. The lack of a standardized definition for ECMO-related infections, differentiation between colonization and infection, and unreliable clinical markers of infection during ECMO make understanding the relationship between infection and outcomes a challenging and not fully clarified task [37]. Regarding the need for post-transplant ECMO, it was higher after 2011 (over 70%), but it is important to note that, in our center, post-transplant ECMO is protocol-mandated for at least 24 h in patients transplanted urgently with ECMO support. This approach is based on the fact that urgent HT with ECMO is associated with higher rates of PGD [38]. Therefore, maintaining ECMO could help preserve hemodynamics and stability in patients during the first few hours post-transplant. As described in the Methodology section, sustained mechanical support was not considered PGD but rather confirmed ventricular dysfunction with an inability to remove ECMO support within the first 24 h post-transplant. PGD occurred in 19% of the entire series, rising to 24% in the latest era. This prevalence is lower than that reported in studies conducted with ECMO in our setting, where prevalence exceeded 30% [21]. PGD is a severe complication and the leading cause of death within the first 30 days after transplantation [31]. It is known that PGD is much more frequent in urgent HT compared to elective cases, and within urgent HT, it is more common in patients arriving for HT with mechanical assistance [39,40]. The likely explanation for the relationship between ECMO assistance and PGD is linked to the systemic effects of ECMO. ECMO support is associated with immunological alterations (increased circulating immature neutrophils, lymphocyte dysfunction, etc.) and leads to elevated levels of pro-inflammatory cytokines, such as interleukins and tumor necrosis factor-alpha [41]. There is a trend observed in the periods from 2011 to 2016 and 2017 to 2023 towards a lower prevalence of renal failure and a higher proportion of patients requiring tracheostomy and reoperation due to bleeding and/or tamponade. The exact reasons for the reduction in renal failure over the years are complex and heterogeneous, involving pre-existing renal disease, acute injury during surgery, and calcineurin inhibitor toxicity. Routine ECMO maintenance in the early hours may have favored renal perfusion and minimized the deleterious effects of surgery and the onset of immunosuppression. The increased need for tracheostomy in recent eras may be influenced by myopathy, the waiting times until an organ is obtained, and pre-transplant mechanical ventilation, as mentioned earlier. Regarding reoperations for bleeding, it should be noted that the exposure of blood to non-biological components of the circuit activates the coagulation system and degrades hemostatic factors [42]. This, coupled with systemic anticoagulation requirements, potential thrombocytopenia, hypofibrinogenemia, and the shear-mediated loss of key platelet surface molecules like selectin and high molecular weight von Willebrand multimers [43], contributes to these complications. Lastly, concerning complications, there is a higher frequency of severe myopathy observed in the periods from 2011 to 2016 and 2017 to 2023, likely due to increased ECMO duration over the years until organ procurement and the impact of mechanical ventilation. Mechanical ventilation, besides being associated with post-transplant morbidity and mortality, reflects a pre-transplant state of myopathy that limits spontaneous ventilation. There is extensive information in the literature regarding complications associated with long-term assist devices from clinical trials and multicenter registries. However, fewer studies have systematically addressed the incidence and clinical impact of complications associated with short-term mechanical circulatory support devices. The high incidence of complications is probably the main drawback of short-term assist devices, and there is evidence that these complications have a significant impact on post-transplant mortality.

Following the analysis of survival and complications, it can be stated that urgent HT with ECMO is a tool that has undoubtedly changed the prognosis of severe HF and urgent HT bridging, offering hopeful survival outcomes for these critically ill patients, albeit with considerable morbidity. The establishment of multidisciplinary teams (ECMO Teams) has allowed for the standardization of processes and appropriate patient selection in this complex scenario [44]. This study has several limitations. Firstly, the number of patients included in the analysis is not high, and they are all from a single center. Secondly, patients with ECMO listed for transplantation who were excluded before the procedure due to multiorgan failure were not considered. Had these patients been transplanted, their mortality and morbidity might have been increased due to their exclusion at the point where transplantation was deemed unfeasible because of multiorgan failure, leading to their subsequent demise. However, the single-center nature of this study ensured a homogeneous and consistent protocol for all patients, likely explaining the absence of differences when comparing different eras. Additionally, it is a series with a sufficient number of cases from a center with extensive experience in cardiac transplantation and ECMO implantation. The prospective nature of this study also lends reliability to the results.

5. Conclusions

VA-ECMO support as a bridge to HT allows discharge from the hospital for three out of every four transplanted patients. This survival rate has remained unchanged over the years. On the other hand, it should be noted that the comorbidities associated with this device are frequent and significant.

Author Contributions: Conceptualization, L.A.B.; methodology, L.A.B. and R.L.-V.; software, L.A.B.; validation, L.A.B. and R.L.-V.; formal analysis, L.A.B.; investigation, L.A.B., B.G.C. and R.L.-V.; resources, L.A.B., B.G.C., S.T.P. and R.L.-V.; data curation, B.G.C., S.T.P. and R.L.-V.; writing—original draft preparation, L.A.B., B.G.C. and R.L.-V.; writing—review and editing, R.L.-V., L.A.B., B.G.C., S.T.P., M.P.G., R.G.C., I.Z.J., F.P.E., P.C., T.H.C., M.T.P., A.P.M., C.D.-M., V.D.T., L.M.D., P.A., Á.C. and J.M.L.; visualization, R.L.-V., L.A.B., B.G.C. and S.T.P.; supervision, L.A.B.; project administration, L.A.B. All authors have read and agreed to the published version of the manuscript.

Funding: This research received no external funding.

Institutional Review Board Statement: The study was conducted in accordance with the Declaration of Helsinki, and approved by the Ethics Committee of Instituto de Investigación Sanitaria La Fe (protocol code ECMO-HF and date of approval 29 May 2024).

Informed Consent Statement: Informed consent was obtained from all subjects involved in this study.

Data Availability Statement: The dataset is available upon request to the authors.

Conflicts of Interest: The authors declare no conflicts of interest.

References

1. Rab, T.; O'Neill, W. Mechanical circulatory support for patients with cardiogenic shock. *Trends Cardiovasc. Med.* **2019**, *29*, 410–417. [CrossRef] [PubMed]
2. López-Vilella, R.; Cervera, B.G.; Trenado, V.D.; Dolz, L.M.; Bonet, L.A. Clinical profiling of patients admitted with acute heart failure: A comprehensive survival analysis. *Front. Cardiovasc. Med.* **2024**, *11*, 1381514. [CrossRef] [PubMed]
3. Martínez-Sellés, M.; Hernández-Pérez, F.J.; Uribarri, A.; Villén, L.M.; Zapata, L.; Alonso, J.J.; Amat-Santos, I.J.; Ariza-Solé, A.; Barrabés, J.A.; Barrio, J.M.; et al. Cardiogenic shock code 2023. Expert document for a multidisciplinary organization that allows quality care. *Rev. Esp. Cardiol. (Engl. Ed.)* **2023**, *76*, 261–269. [CrossRef] [PubMed]

4. Burrell, A.; Kim, J.; Alliegro, P.; Romero, L.; Neto, A.S.; Mariajoseph, F.; Hodgson, C. Extracorporeal membrane oxygenation for critically ill adults. *Cochrane Database Syst. Rev.* **2023**, *2023*, CD010381. [CrossRef]
5. Barge-Caballero, E.; González-Vílchez, F.; Almenar-Bonet, L.; Carmena, M.D.G.-C.; González-Costello, J.; Gómez-Bueno, M.; Castel-Lavilla, M.N.; Lambert-Rodríguez, J.L.; Martínez-Sellés, M.; Mirabet-Pérez, S.; et al. Temporal trends in the use and outcomes of temporary mechanical circulatory support as a bridge to cardiac transplantation in Spain. Final report of the ASIS-TC study. *J. Heart Lung Transplant.* **2023**, *42*, 488–502. [CrossRef]
6. Montisci, A.; Donatelli, F.; Cirri, S.; Coscioni, E.; Maiello, C.; Napoli, C. Veno-arterial Extracorporeal Membrane Oxygenation as Bridge to Heart Transplantation: The Way Forward. *Transplant. Direct.* **2021**, *7*, e720. [CrossRef]
7. Huckaby, L.V.; Hickey, G.; Sultan, I.; Kilic, A. Improvements in Functional Status Among Survivors of Orthotopic Heart Transplantation Following High-risk Bridging Modalities. *Transplantation* **2021**, *105*, 2097–2103. [CrossRef]
8. Sun, H.-Y.; Ko, W.-J.; Tsai, P.-R.; Sun, C.-C.; Chang, Y.-Y.; Lee, C.-W.; Chen, Y.-C. Infections occurring during extracorporeal membrane oxygenation use in adult patients. *J. Thorac. Cardiovasc. Surg.* **2010**, *140*, 1125–1132. [CrossRef]
9. De Prada, J.A.-V.; Arizón, J.M.; Almenar, L.; Vílchez, F.G. Registro Español de Trasplante Cardiaco. *Una Visión Histórica* **2015**, *15*, 27–30.
10. Ariza-Solé, A.; Sánchez-Salado, J.C.; Lorente, V.; González-Costello, J.; Sbraga, F.; Cequier, Á. Learning curve and prognosis in patients with refractory cardiogenic shock receiving ECMO ventricular support. *Med. Intensiva* **2015**, *39*, 523–525.
11. Guilló Moreno, V.; Gutiérrez Martínez, A.; Romero Berrocal, A.; Sánchez Castilla, M.; García-Fernández, J. Experience in the management of ECMO therapy as a mortality risk factor. *Rev. Esp. Anestesiol. Reanim. (Engl. Ed.)* **2018**, *65*, 90–95. [CrossRef] [PubMed]
12. Kobashigawa, J.; Zuckermann, A.; Macdonald, P.; Leprince, P.; Esmailian, F.; Luu, M.; Mancini, D.; Patel, J.; Razi, R.; Reichenspurner, H.; et al. Report from a consensus conference on primary graft dysfunction after cardiac transplantation. *J. Heart Lung Transplant.* **2014**, *33*, 327–340. [CrossRef] [PubMed]
13. Van Diepen, S.; Katz, J.N.; Albert, N.M.; Henry, T.D.; Jacobs, A.K.; Kapur, N.K.; Kilic, A.; Menon, V.; Ohman, E.M.; Sweitzer, N.K.; et al. American Heart Association Coun-cil on Clinical Cardiology; Council on Cardiovascular and Stroke Nursing; Council on Quality of Care and Outcomes Research; and Mission: Lifeline. Contemporary management of cardiogenic shock: A scientific statement from the American Heart Association. *Circulation* **2017**, *136*, e232–e268. [PubMed]
14. Thiele, H.; Jobs, A.; Ouweneel, D.M.; Henriques, J.P.S.; Seyfarth, M.; Desch, S.; Eitel, I.; Pöss, J.; Fuernau, G.; De Waha, S. Percutaneous short-term active mechanical support devices in cardiogenic shock: A systematic review and collaborative meta-analysis of randomized trials. *Eur. Heart J.* **2017**, *38*, 3523–3531. [CrossRef] [PubMed]
15. Thiele, H.; Zeymer, U.; Neumann, F.J.; Ferenc, M.; Olbrich, H.G.; Hausleiter, J. IABP-SHOCK II Trial Investigators. Intraaortic balloon support for myocardial infarction with cardiogenic shock. *N. Engl. J. Med.* **2012**, *367*, 1287–1296. [CrossRef]
16. Stevenson, L.W.; Pagani, F.D.; Young, J.B.; Jessup, M.; Miller, L.; Kormos, R.L.; Naftel, D.C.; Ulisney, K.; Desvigne-Nickens, P.; Kirklin, J.K. INTERMACS Profiles of Advanced Heart Failure: The Current Picture. *J. Heart Lung Transplant.* **2009**, *28*, 535–541. [CrossRef]
17. Pagani, F.D.; Lynch, W.; Swaniker, F.; Dyke, D.B.; Bartlett, R.; Koelling, T.; Moscucci, M.; Deeb, G.M.; Bolling, S.; Monaghan, H.; et al. Extracorporeal life support to left ventricular assist device bridge to heart transplant: A strategy to optimize survival and resource utilization. *Circulation* **1999**, *100*, II206–II210. [CrossRef]
18. Shah, P.; Smith, S.; Haft, J.W.; Desai, S.S.; Burton, N.A.; Romano, M.A.; Aaronson, K.D.; Pagani, F.D.; Cowger, J.A. Clinical outcomes of advanced heart failure patients with cardiogenic shock treated with temporary circulatory support before durable LVAD implant. *ASAIO J.* **2016**, *62*, 20–27. [CrossRef]
19. DeFilippis, E.M.; Clerkin, K.; Truby, L.K.; Francke, M.; Fried, J.; Masoumi, A.; Garan, A.R.; Farr, M.A.; Takayama, H.; Takeda, K.; et al. ECMO as a Bridge to Left Ventricular Assist Device or Heart Transplantation. *JACC Heart Fail.* **2021**, *9*, 281–289. [CrossRef]
20. Fukuhara, S.; Takeda, K.; Kurlansky, P.A.; Naka, Y.; Takayama, H. Extracorporeal membrane oxygenation as a direct bridge to heart transplantation in adults. *J. Thorac. Cardiovasc. Surg.* **2018**, *155*, 1607–1618. [CrossRef]
21. Barge-Caballero, E.; Almenar-Bonet, L.; Gonzalez-Vilchez, F.; Lambert-Rodríguez, J.L.; González-Costello, J.; Segovia-Cubero, J.; Castel-Lavilla, M.A.; Delgado-Jiménez, J.; Garrido-Bravo, I.P.; Rangel-Sousa, D.; et al. Clinical outcomes of temporary mechanical circulatory support as a direct bridge to heart transplantation: A nationwide Spanish registry. *Eur. J. Heart Fail.* **2018**, *20*, 178–186. [CrossRef] [PubMed]
22. Bradbrook, K.; Goff, R.R.; Lindblad, K.; Daly, R.C.; Hall, S. A national assessment of one-year heart outcomes after the 2018 adult heart allocation change. *J. Heart Lung Transplant.* **2023**, *42*, 196–205. [CrossRef] [PubMed]
23. López-Vilella, R.; Sánchez-Lázaro, I.; Moncho, A.P.; Esteban, F.P.; Guillén, M.P.; Jáuregui, I.Z.; Costa, R.G.; Dolz, L.M.; Puerta, S.T.; Bonet, L.A. Complications After Heart Transplantation According to the Type of Pretransplant Circulatory/Ventricular Support. *Transplant. Proc.* **2021**, *53*, 2739–2742. [CrossRef] [PubMed]
24. Barge-Caballero, G.; Castel-Lavilla, M.A.; Almenar-Bonet, L.; Garrido-Bravo, I.P.; Delgado, J.F.; Rangel-Sousa, D.; González-Costello, J.; Segovia-Cubero, J.; Farrero-Torres, M.; Lambert-Rodríguez, J.L.; et al. Venoarterial extracorporeal membrane oxygenation with or without simultaneous intra-aortic balloon pump support as a direct bridge to heart transplantation: Results from a nationwide Spanish registry. *Interact. Cardiovasc. Thorac. Surg.* **2019**, *29*, 670–677. [CrossRef] [PubMed]

25. Rivinius, R.; Helmschrott, M.; Ruhparwar, A.; Erbel, C.; Gleissner, C.A.; Darche, F.F.; Thomas, D.; Bruckner, T.; Katus, H.A.; Doesch, A.O. The influence of surgical technique on early posttransplant atrial fibrillation comparison of biatrial, bicaval, and total orthotopic heart transplantation. *Ther. Clin. Risk Manag.* **2017**, *13*, 287–297. [CrossRef]
26. Morgan, J.A.; Edwards, N.M. Orthotopic cardiac transplantation: Comparison of outcome using biatrial, bicaval, and total techniques. *J. Card. Surg.* **2005**, *20*, 102–106. [CrossRef]
27. Rousse, N.; Juthier, F.; Pinon, C.; Hysi, I.; Banfi, C.; Robin, E.; Fayad, G.; Jegou, B.; Prat, A.; Vincentelli, A. ECMO as a bridge to decision: Recovery, VAD, or heart transplantation? *Int. J. Cardiol.* **2015**, *187*, 620–627. [CrossRef]
28. Moonsamy, P.; Axtell, A.L.; Ibrahim, N.E.; Funamoto, M.; Tolis, G.; Lewis, G.D.; D'alessandro, D.A.; Villavicencio, M.A. Survival after heart transplantation in patients bridged with mechanical circulatory support. *J. Am. Coll. Cardiol.* **2020**, *75*, 2892–2905. [CrossRef]
29. Lui, C.; Fraser, C.D., 3rd; Suarez-Pierre, A.; Zhou, X.; Higgins, R.S.D.; Zehr, K.J.; Choi, C.W.; Kilic, A. Evaluation of extracorporeal membrane oxygenation therapy as a bridging method. *Ann. Thorac. Surg.* **2020**, *112*, 68–74. [CrossRef]
30. Kowalewski, M.; Zieliński, K.; Gozdek, M.; Raffa, G.M.; Pilato, M.; Alanazi, M.; Gilbers, M.; Heuts, S.; Natour, E.; Bidar, E.; et al. Veno-Arterial Extracorporeal Life Support in Heart Transplant and Ventricle Assist Device Centres. Meta-analysis. *ESC Heart Fail.* **2021**, *8*, 1064–1075. [CrossRef]
31. González-Vílchez, F.; Hernández-Pérez, F.; Almenar-Bonet, L.; Crespo-Leiro, M.G.; López-Granados, A.; Ortiz-Bautista, C.; Delgado-Jiménez, J.F.; de Antonio-Ferrer, M.; Sobrino-Márquez, J.M.; García-Romero, E. Spanish Heart Transplant Teams. Spanish heart transplant registry. 34th official report of the Heart Failure Association of the Spanish Society of Cardiology. *Rev. Esp. Cardiol. Engl. Ed.* **2023**, *76*, 901–909. [CrossRef] [PubMed]
32. Bidar, F.; Lancelot, A.; Lebreton, G.; De Chambrun, M.P.; Schmidt, M.; Hékimian, G.; Juvin, C.; Bréchot, N.; Schoell, T.; Leprince, P.; et al. Venous or arterial thromboses after venoarterial extracorporeal membrane oxygenation support: Frequency and risk factors. *J. Heart Lung Transplant.* **2021**, *40*, 307–315. [CrossRef] [PubMed]
33. Cevasco, M.R.; Li, B.; Han, J.; Chiuzan, C.; Mauro, C.M.; Kurlansky, P.; Garan, A.R.; Takeda, K.; Naka, Y.; Takayama, H. Adverse Event Profile Associated with Prolonged Use of CentriMag Ventricular Assist Device for Refractory Cardiogenic Shock. *ASAIO J.* **2019**, *65*, 806–811. [CrossRef] [PubMed]
34. Abrams, D.; Grasselli, G.; Schmidt, M.; Mueller, T.; Brodie, D. ECLS-associated infections in adults: What we know and what we dont yet know. *Intensive Care Med.* **2020**, *46*, 182–191. [CrossRef] [PubMed]
35. Solla-Buceta, M.; González-Vílchez, F.; Almenar-Bonet, L.; Lambert-Rodríguez, J.L.; Segovia-Cubero, J.; González-Costello, J.; Delgado, J.F.; Pérez-Villa, F.; Crespo-Leiro, M.G.; Rangel-Sousa, D.; et al. Infectious complications associated with short-term mechanical circulatory support in urgent heart transplant candidates. *Rev. Espanola Cardiol.* **2022**, *75*, 141–149. [CrossRef]
36. Grasselli, G.; Scaravilli, V.; Di Bella, S.; Biffi, S.; Bombino, M.; Patroniti, N.; Bisi, L.; Peri, A.M.; Pesenti, A.; Gori, A.; et al. Nosocomial infections during extracorporeal membrane oxygenation: Incidence, etiology, and impact on patients outcome. *Crit. Care Med.* **2017**, *45*, 1726–1733. [CrossRef]
37. Marinoni, M.; Migliaccio, M.L.; Trapani, S.; Bonizzoli, M.; Gucci, L.; Cianchi, G.; Gallerini, A.; Buoninsegni, L.T.; Cramaro, A.; Valente, S.; et al. Cerebral microemboli detected by transcranial Doppler in patients treated with extracorporeal membrane oxygenation. *Acta Anaesthesiol. Scand.* **2016**, *60*, 934–944. [CrossRef]
38. Singh, S.S.M.A.; Banner, N.R.; Rushton, S.M.; Simon, A.R.; Berry, C.; Al-Attar, N.P. ISHLT Primary Graft Dysfunction Incidence, Risk Factors, and Outcome: A UK National Study. *Transplantation* **2019**, *103*, 336–343. [CrossRef]
39. López-Vilella, R.; Sánchez-Lázaro, I.J.; Cabanes, M.P.F.; Moncho, A.P.; Bertolín, L.D.; Costa, R.G.; Puigdollers, I.M.; Dolz, L.M.; Jauregui, I.Z.; Puerta, S.T.; et al. Influence of the Type of Circulatory/Ventricular Assistance in the Primary Graft Failure and Heart Transplantation Mortality. *World J. Cardiovasc. Dis.* **2019**, *9*, 545–552. [CrossRef]
40. Carmena, M.D.G.C.; Bueno, M.G.; Almenar, L.; Delgado, J.F.; Arizón, J.M.; Vilchez, F.G.; Crespo-Leiro, M.G.; Mirabet, S.; Roig, E.; Villa, F.P.; et al. Primary graft failure after heart transplantation: Characteristics in a contemporary cohort and performance of the radial risk score. *J. Heart Lung Transplant.* **2013**, *32*, 1187–1195. [CrossRef]
41. Frerou, A.; Lesouhaitier, M.; Gregoire, M.; Uhel, F.; Gacouin, A.; Reizine, F.; Moreau, C.; Loirat, A.; Maamar, A.; Nesseler, N.; et al. Venoarterial extracorporeal membrane oxygenation induces early immune alterations. *Crit. Care.* **2021**, *25*, 9. [CrossRef] [PubMed]
42. Doyle, A.J.; Hunt, B.J. Current understanding of how extracorporeal membrane oxygenators activate haemostasis and other blood components. *Front. Med.* **2018**, *5*, 352. [CrossRef] [PubMed]
43. Olson, S.R.; Murphree, C.R.; Zonies, D.; Meyer, A.D.; Mccarty, O.J.T.; Deloughery, T.G.; Shatzel, J.J. Thrombosis and bleeding in extracorporeal membrane oxygenation (ECMO) without anticoagulation: A systematic review. *ASAIO J.* **2021**, *67*, 290–296. [CrossRef] [PubMed]
44. DellaVolpe, J.; Barbaro, R.P.; Cannon, J.W.; Fan, E.; Greene, W.R.M.; Gunnerson, K.J.M.; Napolitano, L.M.M.; Ovil, A.; Pamplin, J.C.M.; Schmidt, M.; et al. Joint Society of Critical Care Medicine-Extracorporeal Life Support Organization Task Force Position Paper on the role of the intensivist in the initiation and management of extracorporeal membrane oxygenation. *Crit. Care Med.* **2020**, *48*, 838–846. [CrossRef]

biomedicines

MDPI

Article

Exercise-Induced Proteomic Profile Changes in Patients with Advanced Heart Failure

Anna Drohomirecka [1,*], Joanna Waś [2], Ewa Sitkiewicz [3], Bianka Świderska [3], Anna Lutyńska [2], Tomasz Rywik [1] and Tomasz Zieliński [1]

1 Department of Heart Failure and Transplantation, National Institute of Cardiology, Alpejska 42, 04-628 Warsaw, Poland; tzielinski@ikard.pl (T.Z.)
2 Department of Medical Biology, National Institute of Cardiology, Alpejska 42, 04-628 Warsaw, Poland
3 Mass Spectrometry Laboratory, Institute of Biochemistry and Biophysics, Polish Academy of Sciences, 5a Pawinski Street, 02-106 Warsaw, Poland; ewa@ibb.waw.pl (E.S.)
* Correspondence: adrohomirecka@ikard.pl

Abstract: Background/Objectives: The pathophysiological background of the processes activated by physical activity in patients with heart failure (HF) is not fully understood. Proteomic studies can help to preliminarily identify new protein markers for unknown or poorly defined physiological processes. We aimed to analyse the changes in the plasma proteomic profile of HF patients after a cardiopulmonary exercise test (CPET) to define pathways involved in the response to exercise. Methods: The study prospectively enrolled 20 male patients with advanced HF (aged 53.3 $\pm$ 8.3 years). Blood samples were taken from the patients before and immediately after the CPET to obtain plasma proteomic profiles. Two-sample *t*-tests (paired or non-paired) were performed with and without false discovery rate (FDR) correction for multiple testing. Enrichment analysis was performed to associate biological processes and pathways with the study results. Results: A total of 968 plasma proteins were identified, of which 722 underwent further statistical analysis. Of these, 236 proteins showed differential expression when comparing all plasma samples collected before and after CPT ($p < 0.05$), and for 86 of these the difference remained statistically significant after FDR correction. Proteins whose expression changed after exercise are mostly involved in immune response and inflammatory processes, coagulation, cell adhesion, regulation of cellular response to stimulus and regulation of programmed cell death. There were no differences in resting proteomics according to HF etiology (ischemic vs. non-ischemic). Conclusions: Changes in the proteomic profile revealed a complexity of exercise-induced processes in patients with HF, suggesting that few major physiological pathways are involved. Further studies focusing on specific pathways are needed.

Keywords: heart failure; exercise intolerance; proteomic profile; exerkines

1. Introduction

Heart failure (HF) affects 1–2% of adults in developed countries [1]. Despite the continuous development of medical therapies, HF remains a condition with a poor prognosis, associated with significant impairment of quality of life.

HF is not a single pathological diagnosis. Nonetheless, regardless of its etiology, all HF cases are characterized by elevated intracardiac pressures and/or inadequate cardiac output at rest and/or during exercise [1]. Furthermore, as a clinical syndrome, chronic HF is accompanied by typical signs and symptoms, of which exercise intolerance with muscle fatigue and dyspnea is always a hallmark. Although hemodynamic alternations with impaired cardiac reserve followed by reduced peripheral and respiratory skeletal muscle perfusion are an underlying mechanism of impaired exercise capacity in HF, many other factors contribute. Poor pump function activates numerous neurohumoral effects that modify the physiological processes in the peripheral systems. Phillips et al. [2] described contributors to exercise limitation in HF, stressing the role of impaired metabolic vasodilation of exercising muscles. The following have been mentioned as potential mechanisms leading to enhanced vasoconstrictor tone and, consequently, to decreased tissue perfusion: increased sympathetic nervous system activation, activation of the renin–angiotensin system, impaired endothelial-dependent vasodilation, reduced blood vessel density, and increased arterial stiffness [2]. The skeletal muscles per se are also involved in the pathophysiology of HF. Several anatomical and biochemical features have been defined in the course of HF-related skeletal myopathy [3], of which mitochondrial dysfunction is responsible for the majority of the reduced energy supply [3]. Another key player in exercise intolerance in patients with HF are disturbances in respiratory system functioning due to perfusion and ventilation abnormalities [2]. Pulmonary edema (including subclinical fluid retention), increased pulmonary pressure and vascular resistance, decreased elastic recoil of the lungs, inspiratory muscle weakness, and ventilation–perfusion mismatch—all jeopardize gas exchange and oxygen utilization by the mitochondria [2,3].

The above mentioned processes show how complex the interrelationships are between the various organs and systems involved in response to physical activity. Many of them are still not yet fully understood. Numerous cells and tissues secrete signaling moiety in response to acute exercise. Exercise-induced peptides, metabolites, DNA, mRNA, microRNA and other RNA species that exhibit autocrine, paracrine and/or endocrine activity are collectively referred to as exerkines [4]. The last few years have brought new insights into exerkine research with important contributions from "omics" technology [5–8] revealing a broad spectrum of plasma proteome changes after acute exercise compared to rest. However, to the best of our knowledge, no published studies have addressed plasma proteome kinetics in patients with HF as a result of physical exertion.

Therefore, the aim of the current study was to investigate whether there are large-scale plasma proteomic changes in patients with advanced HF after acute extensive exercise and to to define the pathways involved in response to exercise.

2. Material and Methods

2.1. Study Population and Design

2.1.1. Patients

This is a prospective study conducted at a tertiary cardiology center.

The study group consisted of 20 male patients with advanced chronic HF admitted to our center for an evaluation of heart transplant candidacy.

We randomly selected 10 men with ischemic and 10 men with non-ischemic etiologies of HF from a population of 51 patients examined in our earlier study [9], the inclusion criteria of which were: patients aged 18–70 years with advanced heart failure with reduced left ventricular ejection fraction (LVEF; less than 40%) who have clinical indication to undergo a cardiopulmonary exercise test (CPET) and right heart catheterization. Therefore, the exclusion criteria were as previously described [9]: administration of catecholamines, contraindications to performance of CPET, pneumonia or bronchitis within last two weeks, or severe ventilation disorders with forced expiratory volume in one second (FEV1) < 50%.

2.1.2. Cardiopulmonary Exercise Test [9] (As Described Previously)

Symptom-limited submaximal CPET was performed in all patients as a part of diagnostic process and was used to estimate exercise capacity. Peak oxygen consumption was measured with a CPET on a bicycle ergometer (product of Lode Medical Technology, Groningen, The Netherlands). System calibration was performed prior to each test. The exercise test consisted of three minutes of unloaded pedaling followed by a graded increase in workload of 10 watts per minute. All tests were stopped at the request of the patients on the basis of their symptoms (severe dyspnea or fatigue). Peak VO2 was defined as the highest 30-s mean value during the period immediately before the end of exercise. Age- and sex-adjusted peak VO2 was automatically calculated by the system software (MetaLyzer 3B-R2, Cortex, Leipzig, Germany) After exercise was completed, patients spent at least

2 min in a cool-down period on the bicycle without workload. The expiratory exchange ratio [RER, defined as carbon dioxide output (VCO2) divided by oxygen consumption (VO2)] and VE/VCO2 slope (the relation between minute ventilation and carbon dioxide production) were calculated for diagnostic purposes.

2.1.3. Blood Sampling and Storage

Venous blood samples were collected at rest and after completion of the CPET (after a resting period of 10 to 15 min). Plasma was frozen immediately after centrifugation and stored at −80 °C until analysis.

2.2. Laboratory Methods

2.2.1. Protein Digestion

Internal standard (IS) samples were prepared by mixing equal volumes of plasma from each patient. Samples and IS were immunodepleted of the top 14 plasma proteins using High-Select Top 14 Abundant Protein Depletion Resin (Thermo Fisher Scientific; Waltham, MA, USA) according to the manufacturer's protocol. Protein concentrations were measured using the Pierce™ Quantitative Colorimetric Peptide Assay (Thermo Fisher Scientific, Waltham, MA, USA).

25 µg of protein from each sample and IS was dried in a SpeedVac and reconstituted in a digestion buffer containing 5% trifluoroethanol, 5 mM tris(2-carboxyethyl)phosphine (TCEP) and 100 mM triethylammonium bicarbonate (TEAB). After 1 h incubation at 60 °C, the cysteines were blocked with 10 mM methyl methanethiosulfonate (MMTS). Proteins were digested overnight at 37 °C with 2 µg trypsin (Promega GmbH, Mannheim, Germany). Peptides were labeled with TMTpro 16plex tags (Thermo Fisher Scientific, Waltham, MA, USA) in 40 µL of acetonitrile for 1 h on vortex. Three labeling kits were used for the experiment, with 126 tags used to label the IS sample on each TMTpro set. The reaction was quenched by the addition of 8 µL of 5% hydroxylamine. After checking the labeling efficiency, the peptides were combined within each TMTpro set and desalted using 30 mg Oasis HLB columns (Waters Corporation; Milford, MA, USA). Briefly, the cartridges were preconditioned with 1 mL methanol and washed with 1 mL 1.5% acetonitrile (ACN) and 0.1% formic acid (FA). After sample loading and rinsing with 1 mL 1.5% ACN and 0.1% FA, peptides were eluted from the columns with 400 µL 90% ACN and 0.1% FA. Aliquots were dried in a SpeedVac and resuspended in 500 µL of 10 mM ammonium hydroxide with 2% ACN.

2.2.2. Reversed-Phase Peptide Fractionation at High pH

TMT-labeled peptides were fractionated using high-pH reversed-phase chromatography on an XBridge Peptide BEH C18 column (4.6 × 250 mm, 130 Å, 5 µm, Waters). Separation was performed at a flow rate of 0.8 mL/min for 100 min on a Waters Acquity UPLC H-class system. The mobile phases consisted of water (A), acetonitrile (B) and 100 mM ammonium hydroxide solution (C). The percentage of phase C was maintained at 10% throughout the gradient. Fractions were collected every 1 min starting from the fourth minute of the run. The following gradient was used: 5 to 8% solvent B for 3 min, 8 to 15% for 17 min, 15 to 25% for 25 min, 25 to 33% for 15 min, 33 to 50% for 16 min, 50 to 90% for 8 min, 4 min isocratic hold at 90% and final column equilibration at 3% phase B for 2 min. The peptide elution profile was monitored at 214 nm. A total of 96 fractions were dried in Speedvac and reconstituted in Evosep solvent A (0.1% FA in water) by vortexing and sonication for 30 min each. Samples were concatenated by mixing every 48 fractions.

2.2.3. Mass Spectrometry

Fractions were analyzed using an LC-MS system consisting of an Evosep One (Evosep Biosystems, Odense, Denmark) directly coupled to an Orbitrap Exploris 480 mass spectrometer (Thermo Fisher Scientific, Bremen, Germany). Concatenated peptide fractions were applied to disposable Evotips C18 trap columns (Evosep Biosystems, Odense, Denmark) as previously described [10]. Chromatography was performed at a flow rate of 500 nL/min using the 44 min (30 samples per day) preformed gradient on the EV1106 analytical column (Dr. Maisch C18 AQ, 1.9 µm beads, 150 µm ID, 15 cm long, Evosep Biosystems, Odense, Denmark). Data were acquired in positive mode using a data dependent method with the following parameters: MS1 resolution was set to 60,000 with a normalized AGC target of 300%, auto maximum inject time, and a scan range of 300 to 1700 m/z. For MS2 the resolution was set to 30,000 with a standard normalized AGC target, auto maximum inject time and the top 25 precursors within a 1.2 m/z isolation window were considered for MS/MS analysis. Dynamic exclusion was set to 20 s with a mass tolerance of ± 10 ppm, a precursor intensity threshold of 5×10^3 and a Precursor Fit threshold of 70%. Precursors were fragmented in HCD mode with normalized collision energy of 30%. TurboTMT resolution mode was set to "TMTpro Reagents". Spray voltage was set to 2.1 kV, funnel RF level to 40, and heated capillary temperature to 275 °C.

3. Analytical Methods

3.1. Data Analysis

Offline recalibration, as well as peptide and protein identification, were performed in the MaxQuant/Andromeda software suite (version 2.0.1.0) [11] using the Homo sapiens Swissprot database (version 202208, canonical) and the MaxQuant contaminant database (version 2.0.1.0). The search included tryptic-generated peptides, with Metylthio (C) set as a fixed modification and Oxidation (M) as a variable modification. Reporter MS2 TMTpro 16-plex quantification was specified in order to obtain values for quantitative analysis. The reverse database was used for target/decoy statistical results validation, and peptide and protein FDR was set to 0.01. The isobaric match between runs function was enabled.

Protein groups along with quantitative data were further analyzed in Perseus (version 1.6.15) [12]. Hits from the reverse database, proteins identified only by site, and contaminants were removed. Data were normalized using the loading factor (LF) method. LF coefficients for each TMTpro channel were obtained by dividing the sum of the signal for all samples by the sum of the signal for proteins within a given channel. Intensity values for each protein within a sample were multiplied by the LF factor for that channel. Data were logarithmized, and proteins that were not identified in at least 60% of the samples were removed. The remaining missing data were imputed within the normal distribution of intensity, shifted toward the lowest values. A procedure was then performed to remove the batch effect of the TMT set on the signal intensity for individual samples (remove batch effect, Limma R algorithm). The validity of the procedure was checked using data distributions, Person correlation factors and PCA analysis.

3.2. Protein Identification

A total of 968 plasma proteins were identified, of which 772 were suitable for statistical analysis. The complete list of the 772 proteins that were subjected to analysis can be found in the Supplementary File S1.

3.3. Statistical Analysis

Two-sample *t*-tests were used to compare differences between continuous variables (paired or non-paired, as appropriate). The tests were performed with and without false discovery rate (FDR) correction for multiple testing.

3.4. Gene Enrichment Analysis

Gene-encoding proteins identified as significantly altered (with FDR correction) in response to CPET were selected for enrichment analysis to link them to underlying molecular pathways and functional categories defined by gene ontology (GO). Enrichment analysis was performed with the 0.80 version of ShinyGO®—a web application http://bioinformatics.sdstate.edu/go/) (accessed on 1 June 2024) [13].

4. Results

The mean age of the patients was 53.3 ± 8.3 years (range 36 to 64 years). All patients presented with heart failure with reduced ejection fraction (HFrEF) and advanced symptoms (New York Heart Association (NYHA) functional class II–III).

Pharmacological treatment was prescribed according to the European Society of Cardiology guidelines in force at the time of enrollment.

Table 1 provides further details on patient characteristics.

A comparison of pre- and post-exercise plasma samples yielded 236 differential proteins ($p < 0.05$), of which 86 proteins met the criterion after correction for multiple testing.

Table 1. Clinical characteristics of the study population. ACEI = angiotensin-converting enzyme inhibitor, ARB = angiotensin receptor blocker, ARNI = angiotensin receptor-neprylisin inhibitor, COPD = chronic obstructive pulmonary disease, CRT-D = cardiac resynchronization therapy defibrillator, eGFR = estimated glomerular filtration rate, HF = heart failure, ICD = implantable cardioverter defibrillator, LVEDD = left ventricular end-diastolic dimension, LVEF = left ventriclar ejection fraction, NYHA = New York Heart Association, MRA = mineralocorticoid receptor antagonist, NT-pro-BNP = N-terminal prohormone of brain natriuretic peptide, pVO2 = peak oxygen uptake, RER = respiratory exchange ratio, TAPSE = tricuspid annular plane systolic excursion, VE/VCO_2 = minute ventilation/carbon dioxide production * mitral or tricuspidal regurgitation at least moderate.

	Study Population (n = 20)
Clinical characteristics	
Age, years	53.3 ± 8.3
Gender, % male	20 (100)
Ischemic etiology of HF	10 (50)
Atrial fibrillation	11 (55)
Hypertension	7 (35)
Diabetes mellitus	9 (45)
COPD	2 (10)
ICD/CRT-D	12 (60)/6 (30)
II NYHA class, patients (%)	1 (5)
II/III NYHA class, patients (%)	4 (20)
III NYHA class, patients (%)	15 (75)
Echocardiographic parameters	
LVEF [%]	22.2 ± 6.2 (range:12.5–35%)
LVEDD [mm]	73.5 ± 9.6
TAPSE [mm]	18.4 ± 2.4
Mitral regurgitation *, patients (%)	15 (75)
Tricuspid regurgitation *, patients (%)	10 (50)
Laboratory test results	
NT-pro-BNP [pg/mL], median (interquartile range)	3187 (2011–4887)
eGFR, mL/min/1.73 m^2	60.1 ± 14.1
bilirubin [mmol/L]	22.4 ± 11.7
Medication	
Beta-blockers [n, %]	20 (100.0)

Table 1. *Cont.*

	Study Population (n = 20)
ACEI/ARB/ARNI [n, %]	20 (100.0)
Spironolactone/eplerenone [n, %]	20 (100)
Loop diuretics [n, %]	20 (100)
More than one diuretic administered (except from MRA) [n, %]	10 (50)
Cardiopulmonary exercise test results	
pVO2 [mL/kg/min]	10.5 ± 3.3
pVO2 adjusted for sex and age adjusted pVO2 [%]	34.5 ± 10.9
RER at peak exhaustion	1.1 ± 0.1
VE/VCO$_2$ slope	45.2 ± 11.3

Comparison of post- CPET to pre-CPET samples in patients with ischemic etiology of HF yielded 215 differential proteins ($p < 0.05$) of which 22 were found after FDR correction (q < 0.05). For the remaining comparisons (listed below), no proteins were found that met the criterion for statistical significance after adjustment for multiple testing.

When comparing post-CPET vs. pre-CPET samples in patients with non-ischemic etiology of HF, 66 differential proteins were detected. Pre-CPET samples from patients with ischemic vs. non-ischemic etiology differed in 45 proteins, and post-CPET samples differed in 14 proteins between these groups ($p < 0.05$).

For a detailed list of the identified proteins, including the differential proteins, see the Supplementary File S1.

Enrichment Analysis

Detailed data are shown in the Supplementary File S1 and presented as graphs, divided into three types of analyses regarding molecular function, biological process, cellular component (Figures 1–3; (http://bioinformatics.sdstate.edu/go/) accessed on 1 June 2024 [13]) and interactive enrichment network graph (Figure 4, (http://bioinformatics.sdstate.edu/go/://bioinformatics.sdstate.edu/go/) accessed on 1 June 2024 [13]).

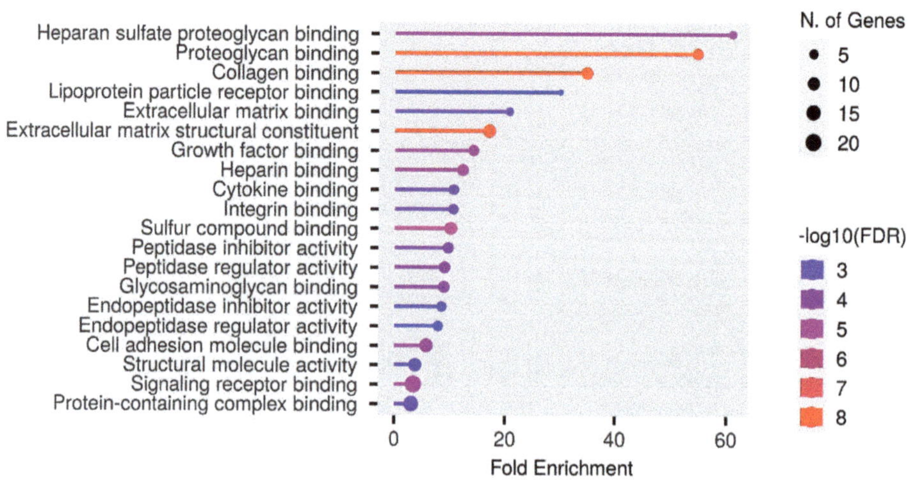

Figure 1. Enrichment analysis: molecular function.

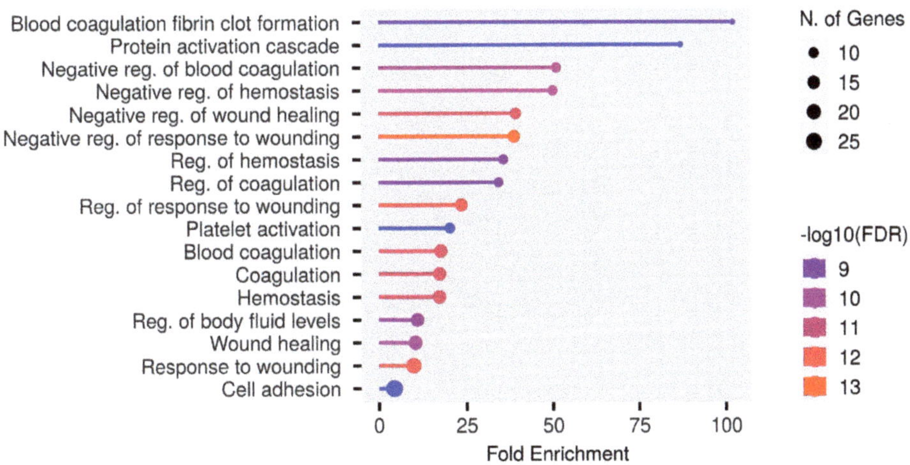

Figure 2. Enrichment analysis: biological processes.

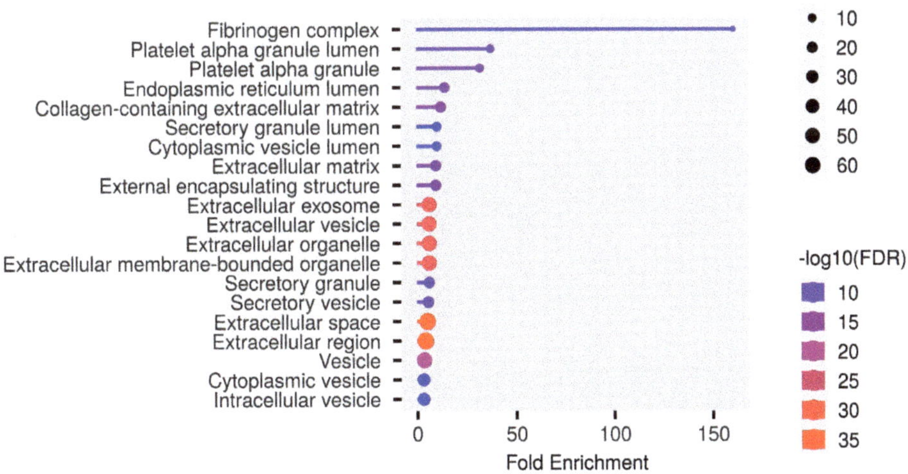

Figure 3. Enrichment analysis: cellular component.

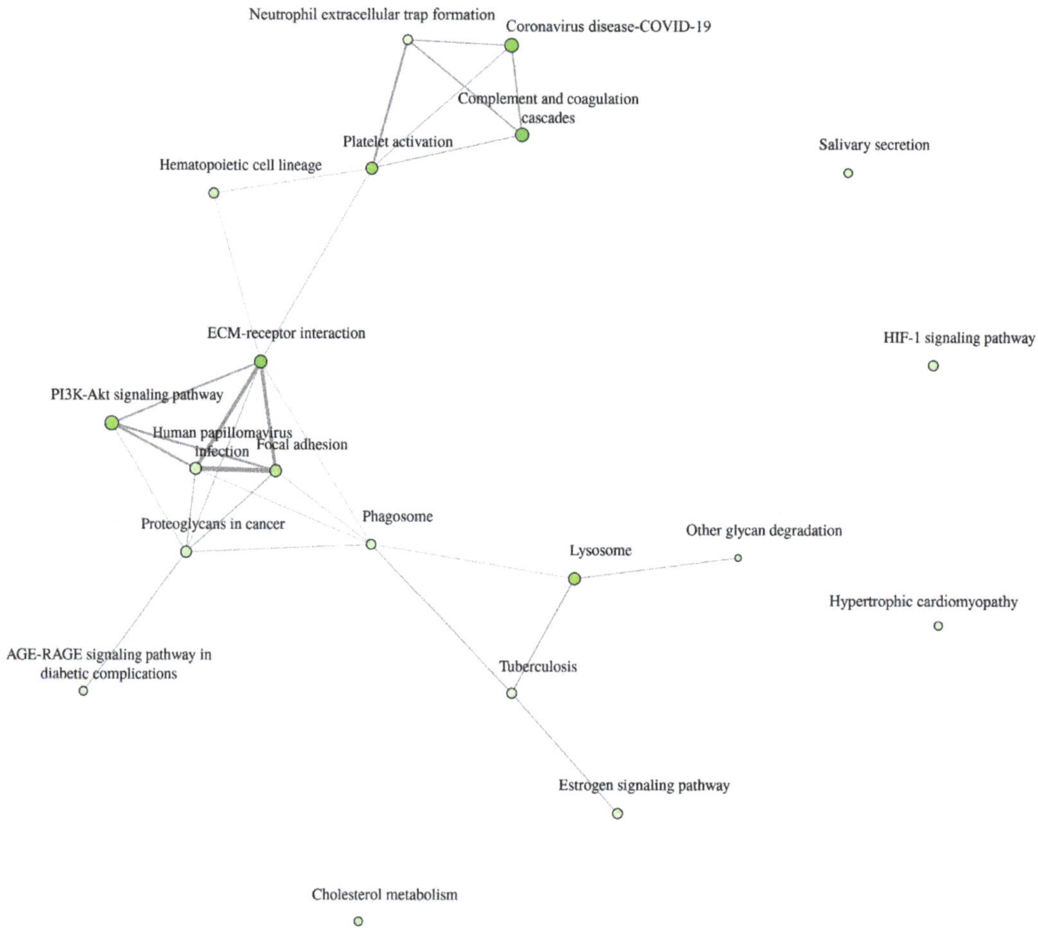

Figure 4. Interactive enrichment network.

5. Discussion

Acute exercise results in an extensive effort of multiple organs and regulations systems, involving not only the skeletal muscle and cardiopulmonary system, but also the neural and endocrine systems. Previous studies [5–7] have showed a broad spectrum of changes in plasma proteome provoked by a single bout of exercise. In designing our study, we had to address some important methodological issues that could significantly affect the results. The first was to determine the optimal time to collect a blood sample after exercise. As shown by Mi et al. [6], the change in the proteome induced by exercise decreases with time, and one hour after peak exercise only 7% of the proteins still present a changed expression. At the same time, new sets of proteins with altered expression are discovered, but they are not as numerous. Because we wanted to define the response to acute exercise in HF patients, we decided to take blood samples during the resting period, no later than 15 min after completion of the CPT. In this way, we minimized the risk of unanticipated injury associated with needle punctures (this can happen when taking blood while exercising or while standing) and were able to detect the majority of proteomic changes. The second issue is natural fluctuations in the proteome. Contrepois et al. [5] compared changes observed after symptom-limited cardiopulmonary exercise with changes observed in individuals without intervention in 1-h and 24-h windows. They concluded that less than 2% of the analytes that changed with exercise also varied within an hour without exercise, but usually with a different magnitude or trajectory. In addition, they found that exercise-induced changes were significantly more pronounced (at least 2-fold greater) than individual spontaneous inter-day variation within 24 h. These findings support our assumption that the natural intra-personal variability of the proteome may be marginalized in the context of exercise-induced changes. Moreover, we included patients who were clinically stable with no symptoms of worsening HF to reduce the risk that the observed results were a consequence of disease exacerbation. Finally, our concern was the size of the study population. Proteomic studies have been performed on even smaller samples (e.g., 12 individuals [7], six men [8]) and such a group size is acceptable. We tried to select a more homogeneous population rather than a large one, especially since it has been shown that the inter-individual variability in response to an acute bout of exercise was more evident for proteins than, for example, for metabolites or transcripts [5].

In our study, 86 proteins were found to be differentially expressed after CPET (after correction for multiple testing). This number is lower than that observed in most studies in subjects without heart failure [5–7], although Kurgan et al. [8] identified only 20 proteins whose expression changed after acute exercise. There is no simple explanation for such a large difference between studies. In the case of our population, a smaller number of differential proteins may be related to the intensity of the exercise performed by the patients. Guseh et al. [7] found that although most proteins that changed their expression after moderate intensity exercise remained over- or under-expressed after high intensity exercise, the number of differential proteins increased significantly (from 184 to 598) with increasing exercise intensity. The individuals enrolled in the previous studies were of normal physical capacity. In contrast, we focused on patients with significant exercise intolerance due to heart failure—all study participants were classified as at least New York Heart Association II class and were only able to achieve approximately 35% of the predicted peak oxygen consumption.

Enrichment analysis of our results showed the strongest correlation of the differential proteins with regulation of coagulation/homeostasis, wound healing, protein activation cascade, body fluid levels and cell adhesion. Particularly noteworthy is the discussion of proteins involved in the regulation of coagulation processes. Changes in the expression of procoagulant and fibrinolytic proteins were observed in studies of subjects without heart failure [5,6], but in patients with heart failure (our study population) they dominated the results of the enrichment analysis. Acute exercise increased fibrinolysis in healthy individuals in a manner dependent on the intensity and duration of the exercise [14]. Furthermore, the fibrinolytic response to exercise seemed to be similar in patients with cardiovascular disease [14]. However, patients with cardiovascular disease showed an increased coagulation potential both at rest and after exercise compared to healthy subjects, involving elevated thrombin–antithrombin complexes and von Willebrand factor [14]. In our study, we observed a significant upregulation of proteins with procoagulant properties, such as von Willebrand factor (similar to the results presented previously [5,6]), fibrinogen, and coagulation factor XII; but surprisingly, at the same time, other procoagulants such as thrombospondin-1 (which has been shown to increase in individuals without heart failure [6]) or coagulation factor XI were downregulated. In addition, we also demonstrated an elevated expression of platelet glycoprotein V. This may indicate that acute, intense exercise increases prothrombotic activity in patients with heart failure, but the extent and consequences of this effect should be further defined. Moreover, Mi et al. [6] found that there was no impact on coagulation during peak exercise as opposed to 1 h after exercise. This suggests that changes in coagulation pathways occur during the recovery period, which is consistent with our results.

An interesting finding showed an interactive enrichment network. It revealed that the PI3K-Akt pathway is involved in the response to intense exercise in HF patients. One of the proteins associated with the PI3K-Akt pathway is interleukin-6. It plays a dual role in inflammatory processes—depending on how it binds to its receptor, it can have proinflammatory or anti-inflammatory effects [15]. The soluble receptor (sIL-6R), upon binding interleukin-6, is capable of inducing intracellular signaling via gp130, referred to as IL-6 trans-signaling, and does not require the presence of Il-6R on the cell membrane [15]. Trans-signaling is responsible for proinflammatory response. In addition, Zegeye et al. [15] showed that Il-6R trans-signaling activates the JAK/STAT3 pathway, along with activation of the PI3K/AKT and MEK/ERK pathways. In turn, Ouwerkerk et al. [16] recently published the results of an analysis of the BIOSTAT-CHF (Systems BIOlogy Study to TAilored Treatment in Chronic Heart Failure) study data using a specifically designed machine learning approach, where they described that 4 major pathways were associated with all-cause mortality in HF patients: (1) the PI3K/Akt pathway; (2) the MAPK pathway; (3) the Ras pathway; and (4) epidermal growth factor receptor tyrosine kinase inhibitor resistance. All of the above indicate that the decrease in interleukin-6 receptor subunit alfa after exercise in HF patients found in our study is not just a coincidental finding, but an expression of real pathophysiological processes.

It is noteworthy that there was a change in the expression of C1q and tumor necrosis factor-related protein 1 (CTRP1), which has been the subject of rather limited study thus far in the context of HF. Yang et al. [17] demonstrated that the levels of CTRP1 in the plasma and epicardial adipose tissue were elevated in patients with heart failure (HF) relative to control subjects. Higher CTRP1 levels were identified as a predictor of a worse prognosis (composite end point: cardiac death and readmission for worsening of heart failure). Furthermore, the experimental model of cell culture demonstrated that CTRP1 increases the release of aldosterone and interleukin 6. The increased expression of CTRP1 following exercise may contribute to the initiation and propagation of inflammatory processes and the activity of the renin–angiotensin system.

5.1. Clinical Implications

One of the primary symptoms of heart failure is exercise intolerance. The prescription of appropriate levels of physical activity, and the selection of appropriate forms of exercise within those levels, represents an inherently complex issue in the management of patients with HF. While excessive physical activity may potentially exacerbate the symptoms of HF, regular physical training has been demonstrated to enhance the quality of life and reduce cardiovascular and all-cause hospitalizations [3,18]. Both European [1] and American guidelines [19] recommend exercise training for clinically stable patients. Nevertheless, there is currently no single training protocol that is dedicated to HF patients with reduced LVEF. The parameters, such as frequency, intensity, duration, type, volume, and progression of training, should be tailored to the individual patient [18]. The proteomic analysis of plasma conducted as part of our study revealed a multitude of alterations in protein expression patterns following CPET in patients with HF. An enrichment analysis identified some pathways that are typical for exercise-induced microinjury (such as regulation of the response to wounding and healing), which are also observed in healthy individuals [3]. However, more importantly, it linked the observed changes with processes that could potentially impact the clinical outcomes of HF such as coagulation disorder and JAK/STAT3 pathway. A change in the regulation of proteins or pathways associated with poor prognosis in patients with HF in response to an acute bout of exercise (CPET in the study) may be indicative not only of advancement of the HF, but also of overexertion. The proteins that are significantly either up- or downregulated during intensive exercise should be subjected to further investigation as potential markers for monitoring the adjustment of training intensity.

The objective of CPET is for the patient to perform a submaximal exercise. A high exercise load can activate physiological mechanisms that are not expressed under resting conditions. Consequently, the expression of proteins that are predictors of patient prognosis is anticipated to undergo alterations in response to stress conditions. The discovery that the PI3K-Akt pathway plays a role in the response to intense exercise in HF patients provides an illustrative example of the second point. Furthermore, the PI3K-Akt pathway exemplifies the advancement of knowledge regarding biomarkers and pathophysiological mechanisms, ultimately facilitating the development of novel treatment options. Recently, Salubris Biotherapeutics presented the results of a phase 1b clinical trial of JK07—first investigational antibody fusion protein and first selective ErbB4 agonist which consists of an active polypeptide fragment of the human growth factor neuregulin [NRG-1] [20]. In an experimental model, NRG-1 was shown to protect the heart against ischemia/reperfusion injury through a PI3K/Akt-dependent mechanism [21]. The clinical trial [20] revealed a significant improvement of LVEF in patients with HF with reduced LVEF six months following the administration of a single dose of JK07. Further investigation of the drug is planned as a phase 2, randomized, double-blind, placebo-controlled, multiple dose study (NCT06369298).

5.2. *Limitations of the Study*

The study group, although very homogeneous, is relatively small. To confirm the results of the study, further research should be performed on a large population targeting the predefined proteins.

The study samples were collected before the common implementation of flosins and sacubitril/walsartan into the therapy of patients with HF. As there are two groups of drugs that have spectacularly improved the prognosis of patients, their impact on the acute response to exercise in HF patients cannot be excluded.

6. Conclusions

Changes in the proteomic profile revealed a complexity of exercise-induced processes in patients with HF, suggesting that few major physiological pathways are involved. Further studies focusing on specific pathways are needed.

Supplementary Materials: The following supporting information can be downloaded at: https://www.mdpi.com/article/10.3390/biomedicines12102267/s1, xls.file named: Supplementary File S1. Supplementary file contains database of proteins identified for analysis and detailed enrichment analysis data.

Author Contributions: Conceptualization, A.D.; methodology, A.D., J.W., E.S., B.Ś. and A.L.; validation, A.D., J.W., E.S. and B.Ś.; formal analysis, A.D., J.W., E.S., B.Ś., T.R. and T.Z.; investigation, A.D., J.W., E.S., B.Ś. and T.R.; resources, A.D., J.W. and A.L.; data curation, A.D., J.W., E.S. and B.Ś.; writing—original draft preparation, A.D., J.W., E.S. and B.Ś.; writing—review and editing, A.D. and T.R.; visualization, A.D., E.S. and B.Ś.; supervision, A.D. and A.L.; project administration, A.D.; funding acquisition, A.D. All authors have read and agreed to the published version of the manuscript.

Funding: The study was founded from National Science Center grant Miniatura 5 No. 2021/05/X/N27/00056.

Institutional Review Board Statement: The study was conducted in accordance with the Declaration of Helsinki and approved by the Regional Ethics Committee of National Institute of Cardiology (approval number: 1928).

Informed Consent Statement: Informed consent was obtained from all subjects involved in the study.

Data Availability Statement: Data are available in Supplementary File S1 and additional data are available upon request.

Acknowledgments: The abstract of the manuscript was submitted and accepted as a poster presentation at the Heart Failure Congress of the European Society of Cardiology in Lisbon, 11–14 May 2024 [22].

Conflicts of Interest: The authors declare no conflicts of interest. The funders had no role in the design of the study; in the collection, analyses, or interpretation of data; in the writing of the manuscript; or in the decision to publish the results.

References

1. McDonagh, T.A.; Metra, M.; Adamo, M.; Gardner, R.S.; Baumbach, A.; Böhm, M.; Burri, H.; Butler, J.; Čelutkienė, J.; Chioncel, O.; et al. 2021 ESC Guidelines for the diagnosis and treatment of acute and chronic heart failure: Developed by the Task Force for the diagnosis and treatment of acute and chronic heart failure of the European Society of Cardiology (ESC). With the special contribution of the Heart Failure Association (HFA) of the ESC. *Eur. J. Hear. Fail.* **2022**, *24*, 4–131. [CrossRef] [PubMed]
2. Phillips, S.A.; Vuckovic, K.; Cahalin, L.P.; Baynard, T. Defining the System: Contributors to Exercise Limitations in Heart Failure. *Hear. Fail. Clin.* **2015**, *11*, 1–16. [CrossRef] [PubMed]
3. Del Buono, M.G.; Arena, R.; Borlaug, B.A.; Carbone, S.; Canada, J.M.; Kirkman, D.L.; Garten, R.; Rodriguez-Miguelez, P.; Guazzi, M.; Lavie, C.J.; et al. Exercise Intolerance in Patients with Heart Failure: JACC State-of-the-Art Review. *J. Am. Coll. Cardiol.* **2019**, *73*, 2209–2225. [CrossRef] [PubMed]
4. Safdar, A.; Saleem, A.; Tarnopolsky, M.A. The potential of endurance exercise-derived exosomes to treat metabolic diseases. *Nat. Rev. Endocrinol.* **2016**, *12*, 504–517. [CrossRef] [PubMed]
5. Contrepois, K.; Wu, S.; Moneghetti, K.J.; Hornburg, D.; Ahadi, S.; Tsai, M.-S.; Metwally, A.A.; Wei, E.; Lee-McMullen, B.; Quijada, J.V.; et al. Molecular Choreography of Acute Exercise. *Cell* **2020**, *181*, 1112–1130. [CrossRef] [PubMed] [PubMed Central]
6. Mi, M.Y.; Barber, J.L.; Rao, P.; Farrell, L.A.; Sarzynski, M.A.; Bouchard, C.; Robbins, J.M.; Gerszten, R.E. Plasma Proteomic Kinetics in Response to Acute Exercise. *Mol. Cell. Proteom.* **2023**, *22*, 100601. [CrossRef] [PubMed] [PubMed Central]
7. Guseh, J.S.; Churchill, T.W.; Yeri, A.; Lo, C.; Brown, M.; Houstis, N.E.; Aragam, K.G.; Lieberman, D.E.; Rosenzweig, A.; Baggish, A.L. An expanded repertoire of intensity-dependent exercise-responsive plasma proteins tied to loci of human disease risk. *Sci. Rep.* **2020**, *10*, 10831. [CrossRef] [PubMed] [PubMed Central]
8. Kurgan, N.; Noaman, N.; Pergande, M.R.; Cologna, S.M.; Coorssen, J.R.; Klentrou, P. Changes to the Human Serum Proteome in Response to High Intensity Interval Exercise: A Sequential Top-Down Proteomic Analysis. *Front. Physiol.* **2019**, *10*, 362. [CrossRef] [PubMed] [PubMed Central]
9. Drohomirecka, A.; Waś, J.; Wiligórska, N.; Rywik, T.M.; Komuda, K.; Sokołowska, D.; Lutyńska, A.; Zieliński, T. L-arginine and Its Derivatives Correlate with Exercise Capacity in Patients with Advanced Heart Failure. *Biomolecules* **2023**, *13*, 423. [CrossRef] [PubMed] [PubMed Central]
10. Nynca, J.; Malinowska, A.; Świderska, B.; Wiśniewska, J.; Dobosz, S.; Ciereszko, A. Triploidization of rainbow trout affects proteins related to ovary development and reproductive activity. *Aquaculture* **2023**, *565*, 739145. [CrossRef]
11. Tyanova, S.; Temu, T.; Cox, J. The MaxQuant computational platform for mass spectrometry-based shotgun proteomics. *Nat. Protoc.* **2016**, *11*, 2301. [CrossRef] [PubMed]
12. Tyanova, S.; Temu, T.; Sinitcyn, P.; Carlson, A.; Hein, M.Y.; Geiger, T.; Mann, M.; Cox, J. The Perseus computational platform for comprehensive analysis of (prote)omics data. *Nat. Methods* **2016**, *13*, 731. [CrossRef] [PubMed]
13. Ge, S.X.; Jung, D.; Yao, R. ShinyGO: A graphical gene-set enrichment tool for animals and plants. *Bioinformatics* **2020**, *36*, 2628–2629. [CrossRef] [PubMed] [PubMed Central]
14. Womack, C.J.; Nagelkirk, P.R.; Coughlin, A.M. Exercise-Induced Changes in Coagulation and Fibrinolysis in Healthy Populations and Patients with Cardiovascular Disease. *Sports Med.* **2003**, *33*, 795–807. [CrossRef] [PubMed]
15. Zegeye, M.M.; Lindkvist, M.; Fälker, K.; Kumawat, A.K.; Paramel, G.; Grenegård, M.; Sirsjö, A.; Ljungberg, L.U. Activation of the JAK/STAT3 and PI3K/AKT pathways are crucial for IL-6 trans-signaling-mediated pro-inflammatory response in human vascular endothelial cells. *Cell Commun. Signal.* **2018**, *16*, 55. [CrossRef] [PubMed] [PubMed Central]
16. Ouwerkerk, W.; Pereira, J.P.B.; Maasland, T.; Emmens, J.E.; Figarska, S.M.; Tromp, J.; Koekemoer, A.L.; Nelson, C.P.; Nath, M.; Romaine, S.P.; et al. Multiomics Analysis Provides Novel Pathways Related to Progression of Heart Failure. *J. Am. Coll. Cardiol.* **2023**, *82*, 1921–1931. [CrossRef] [PubMed]
17. Yang, Y.; Liu, S.; Zhang, R.-Y.; Luo, H.; Chen, L.; He, W.-F.; Lei, R.; Liu, M.-R.; Hu, H.-X.; Chen, M. Association Between C1q/TNF-Related Protein-1 Levels in Human Plasma and Epicardial Adipose Tissues and Congestive Heart Failure. *Cell. Physiol. Biochem.* **2017**, *42*, 2130–2143. [CrossRef] [PubMed]
18. Taylor, J.L.; Myers, J.; Bonikowske, A.R. Practical guidelines for exercise prescription in patients with chronic heart failure. *Hear. Fail. Rev.* **2023**, *28*, 1285–1296. [CrossRef] [PubMed] [PubMed Central]
19. Heidenreich, P.A.; Bozkurt, B.; Aguilar, D.; Allen, L.A.; Byun, J.J.; Colvin, M.M.; Deswal, A.; Drazner, M.H.; Dunlay, S.M.; Evers, L.R.; et al. 2022 AHA/ACC/HFSA Guideline for the Management of Heart Failure: A Report of the American College of Cardiology/American Heart Association Joint Committee on Clinical Practice Guidelines. *Circulation* **2022**, *145*, e895–e1032; Erratum in *Circulation* **2022**, *145*, e1033. https://doi.org/10.1161/CIR.0000000000001073; Erratum in *Circulation* **2022**, *146*, e185. https://doi.org/10.1161/CIR.0000000000001097; Erratum in *Circulation* **2023**, *147*, e674. https://doi.org/10.1161/CIR.0000000000001142. [CrossRef] [PubMed]
20. SalubrisBio. Salubris Biotherapeutics Presents Positive 6-Month Data from Phase 1b Clinical Trial of JK07 in Late-Breaking Session at The Heart Failure Society of America Annual Meeting 2023. Available online: https://www.salubrisbio.com/2023/10/10/salubris-biotherapeutics-presents-positive-6-month-data-from-phase-1b-clinical-trial-of-jk07-in-late-breaking-session-at-the-heart-failure-society-of-america-annual-meeting-2023/ (accessed on 22 September 2024).

21. Fang, S.J.; Wu, X.S.; Han, Z.H.; Zhang, X.X.; Wang, C.M.; Li, X.Y.; Lu, L.Q.; Zhang, J.L. Neuregulin-1 preconditioning protects the heart against ischemia/reperfusion injury through a PI3K/Akt-dependent mechanism. *Chin. Med. J.* **2010**, *123*, 3597–3604. [PubMed]
22. Drohomirecka, A.; Waś, J.; Sitkiewicz, E.; Świderska, B.; Lutyńska, A.; Rywik, T.; Zieliński, T. Exercise-induced proteomic profile changes in patients with advanced heart failure–A pilot study. In Proceedings of the Heart Failure Congress of the European Society of Cardiology, Lisbon, Portugal, 11–14 May 2024.

biomedicines

MDPI

Article

Evaluation of the Accuracy of Point-of-Care Urine Chloride Measured via Strip Test in Patients with Heart Failure

Mateusz Guzik *, Berenika Jankowiak, Piotr Ponikowski and Jan Biegus

Institute of Heart Diseases, Faculty of Medicine, Wroclaw Medical University, Borowska 213, 50-556 Wroclaw, Poland

* Correspondence: mateuszguzik23@gmail.com

Abstract: Background: In clinical practice, patient self-monitoring is crucial in achieving therapeutic goals in various diseases. In heart failure (HF), it is particularly important due to the increasing role of urine composition. Therefore, we proposed this study to assess the accuracy of urine chloride (uCl^-) assessment via strip test in relation to chloride and sodium (uNa^+) measurements in a gold-standard laboratory method. Methods: Urine samples were collected before administering morning medications. Afterwards, they were analyzed concurrently using the strip test and gold-standard laboratory method. Results: The study cohort comprised 66 patients (82% male, mean age 68 ± 12 years), of whom 65% were diagnosed with HF and 35% without HF. Across the entire cohort, a strong correlation was observed between uCl^- measured by both methods (r = 0.85; $p < 0.001$). However, the strip test was found to underestimate uCl^- relative to the laboratory measurements (mean difference of 18 mmol/L). Furthermore, strong correlations were observed between the methods among patients with HF and without HF (r = 0.88 vs. r = 0.71, respectively; $p < 0.001$ for both), where they presented similar relationship patterns. Interestingly, in patients with a low glomerular filtration rate (eGFR $\leq$ 60 mL/min/1.73 m^2), the correlation between both methods was greater compared to those with high eGFR (>60 mL/min/1.73 m^2) (r = 0.94 vs. r = 0.76, respectively; $p < 0.001$ for both). The relationship between uCl^- from the strip test and uNa^+ from the laboratory measurement was weaker than for uCl^-, but it was significant. Conclusions: These findings suggest that point-of-care strip tests for assessing urinary chloride demonstrate high accuracy and potential utility, particularly in patients with reduced eGFR.

Keywords: heart failure; strip test; urine chloride; urine sodium; self-monitoring

1. Introduction

The effective treatment and management of patients with chronic diseases is only possible when they actively participate in the process. Therefore, awareness of their disease, condition, and the importance of self-assessment is crucial. In addition to easily obtainable clinical parameters like body weight and blood pressure, there is an opportunity to extend self-monitoring to include certain hemodynamic and biochemical analyses [1,2]. Among the various parameters recommended for monitoring in clinical conditions, assessing urine composition can be helpful in certain diseases, especially heart failure (HF). It is well established that routine urine assessment in HF serves as an indicator of diuretic response [3–7]. Evidence suggests that, nowadays, in acute HF, diuretic treatment should be guided by urine sodium concentration [5,8–10]. However, due to the difficulty and impracticality of regular/daily urine biochemical parameter assessment, there are no data on such a method for chronic HF outpatient monitoring. Nevertheless, numerous studies have shown that low concentrations of chloride and sodium in the urine are associated not only with a poor diuretic response, but also with worse long-term outcomes [11–13]. This is reasoned in pathophysiology to be because chloride concentration plays a significant role in the regulation of renal blood flow, glomerular filtration, and ion reabsorption/secretion mechanisms in relation to neurohormonal activity [12,14–17]. Importantly, this could contribute to the development of cardiorenal syndrome, which might result in the deterioration of heart and kidney function, leading to impaired glomerular filtration, reduced urine production, and diminished response to loop diuretics [10]. This could limit the effectiveness of decongestive therapy in acute HF and the maintenance of the euvolemic state in chronic HF [12,14]. Additionally, the administration of high doses of diuretics in outpatients could cause dehydration, thirst, and further kidney injury, which could result in diminished sodium and chloride excretion [18–21]. Therefore, a long-term approach involving strict monitoring of critical parameters, such as chloride or sodium excretion, and adjusting the patient's treatment accordingly may be justified. Strip tests that allow for the evaluation of urine chloride concentration have been evaluated in patients with cerebral salt-wasting syndrome, those on home parenteral nutrition, and those with hyponatremia or dehydration. The results were promising. Thus, our aim was to investigate the chloride concentration in urine using a strip test (as a point-of-care examination) to determine the accuracy of such an approach (in comparison to the gold-standard laboratory method). Additionally, due to the absence of strip tests for urine sodium assessment, we evaluated the relationship between urine chloride (assessed via strip test) and urine sodium laboratory assessments, as the currently most evidenced urine ion.

2. Materials and Methods

The study was a prospective, observational, single-center study conducted among patients hospitalized between April and May 2024 in the Institute of Heart Diseases in Wrocław, Poland. The participants included patients with established diagnoses of chronic heart failure, with stable symptoms over time, as well as patients without a diagnosis of heart failure. Basic clinical, laboratory, and echocardiographic data were collected from each participant. The participants were asked to provide a urine sample for biochemical assessment. First, morning urine samples (20 mL) from the first day of hospitalization were collected from patients before they took their morning medications. Each obtained sample was divided into two identical, sterile containers, where both contained 10 mL of urine, to undergo independent assessments. The samples were assessed in the laboratory to measure the chloride and sodium levels in the urine. Simultaneously, the urine was tested using a strip test (Hach, Quantab). All urine samples were assessed by one single physician to simulate the condition in which the patient would self-assess the urine sample.

According to the instructions, the strip test result was taken once the strip indicated the end of the assessment (the indicator at the top of the strip turned black). All strip test results were evaluated by one investigator, blinded to the laboratory measurement results at the time of evaluation. The values indicated in the strip test (mm) were converted to mmol/L using the scale provided in the test specification. The results obtained from the laboratory assessments and the strip tests were compared using the statistical methods described below. Due to the local laboratory's low limit of sodium and chloride measurement, patients with lower than 20 mmol/L sodium and/or chloride established in the strip test were excluded from the study. Additionally, patients whose tests were not completed according to the test instructions were excluded.

In terms of statistical analysis, due to the lack of prior studies, no evidence-based a priori assumptions regarding correlations and sample size could be made. However, based on power analysis (power: 0.80; alpha: 0.05; assumed correlation coefficient: 0.5), the required sample size was estimated at 29 patients. The quantitative variables were analyzed for normality using the Shapiro–Wilk test. Variables with normal distribution are presented as mean ± standard deviation (SD), while those that did not follow a normal distribution are presented as median [interquartile range (IQR)]. The homogeneity of variance was tested by the Levene test. The differences between subsequent variables with normal distribution were evaluated using the *t*-test. Welch's correction was applied when appropriate. Variables with a distribution other than normal were tested using the Mann–Whitney U test. Differences between qualitative variables were examined using the

Chi-Square test. The Pearson correlation test was used to evaluate correlations between values. The Bland–Altman plot was performed to assess the agreement between two measurement methods by plotting the differences between them against their average. Points close to the mean difference indicate good agreement, while those further from the mean suggest discrepancies. The limits of agreement in the Bland–Altman plots were calculated based on the mean difference of measurements: mean difference ± 1.96 standard deviations. Post hoc tests' power was checked. A graphical presentation of the results was made using GraphPad Prism. The statistical analysis was performed in Statistica 13.

3. Results

3.1. Study Population Characteristics

The analysis included 66 patients, predominantly male (79%), with a mean age of 68 ± 12 years. Among the participants, 65% had been diagnosed with heart failure. The median left ventricle ejection fraction (LVEF) was 50 [30–57]%, and the NT-proBNP concentration was 1583 [274–6480] pg/mL. Additionally, 51% of chronic heart failure patients were taking diuretics, with a median furosemide (or equivalent) dose of 20 [0–60] mg.

The summarized characteristics of the study population are presented in Table 1.

Table 1. General characteristics of population.

Parameter	Value
Age (years)	68 ± 12
Sex—male (N; %)	52 (79%)
HR (beats/min)	71 [63–80]
SBP (mmHg)	123 ± 18
DBP (mmHg)	75 ± 11
MAP (mmHg)	91 ± 11
Hgb (g/dL)	12.8 ± 2
Leukocytes (10^3/uL)	7.47 [5.81–9.85]
Creatinine (mg/dL)	1.08 [0.84–1.68]
eGFR (mL/min/1.73 m^2)	70 ± 31
Urea (mg/dL)	46 [32–73]
NT-proBNP (pg/mL)	1 583 [274–6480]
Serum Na^+ (mmol/L)	141 ± 3
Serum K^+ (mmol/L)	4.4 ± 0.5
LVEF (%)	50 [30–57]
TAPSE (mm)	21 ± 5
Arterial hypertension (N; %)	49 (74%)
Diabetes mellitus (N; %)	35 (53%)
Amyloidosis (confirmed or suspected) (N; %)	2 (3%)
Chronic kidney disease (N; %)	23 (35%)
Chronic diuretics administration (N; %)	34 (52%)
Chronically administered loop diuretic dose (furosemide dose equivalent) (mg)	20 [0–60]
SGLT-2 inhibitors (N; %)	33 (48%)
B-blocker (N; %)	55 (83%)
ACEI/ARB (N; %)	31 (47%)
ARNI (N; %)	8 (12%)
MRA (N; %)	31 (47%)
Acetazolamide (N; %)	0 (0%)
Thiazide diuretics (N; %)	3 (5%)

3.2. The Relationship Between the Value Taken from the Strip Test and the Corresponding Chloride Concentration

The pattern between the value taken from the strip test and the corresponding urine chloride is an exponential shape. It was presented in Figure 1. The equation of the best-fit curve is as follows:

$$uCl = 3.33 \times e^{0.44 \times D} \quad (1)$$

uCl^-—Urine chloride concentration.
D—Value taken from strip test.

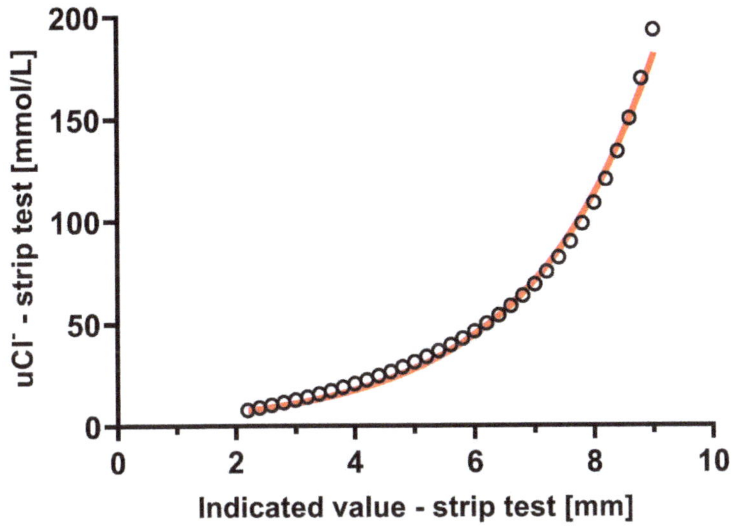

Figure 1. The relationship between corresponding values: the value taken from strip test and corresponding urine chloride concentration according to test specification.

To examine the fit of the curve describing the relationship between the presented values, the relationship was linearized by the logarithmizing the equation:

$$\ln (uCl) = \ln 3.33 \times 0.44 \times D \quad (2)$$

uCl^-—Urine chloride concentration.
D—Value taken from strip test.

For these data R^2 value was 0.998.

3.3. The Relationship Between Urine Chloride Measured in the Laboratory and in the Strip Test

In general, the relationship pattern is linear (with correlation r = 0.85; $p < 0.001$), but the results are dispersed over 40 mmol/L uCl^- with the strip test, especially for higher concentrations of uCl. Nevertheless, discrepancies resulted from the underestimation of uCl in the strip test (laboratory-assessed uCl was, in general, equal to or higher than that measured by the strip test).

Based on a linear regression model, the function of dependence between uCl measured in the laboratory and obtained in the strip test was established (Figure 2).

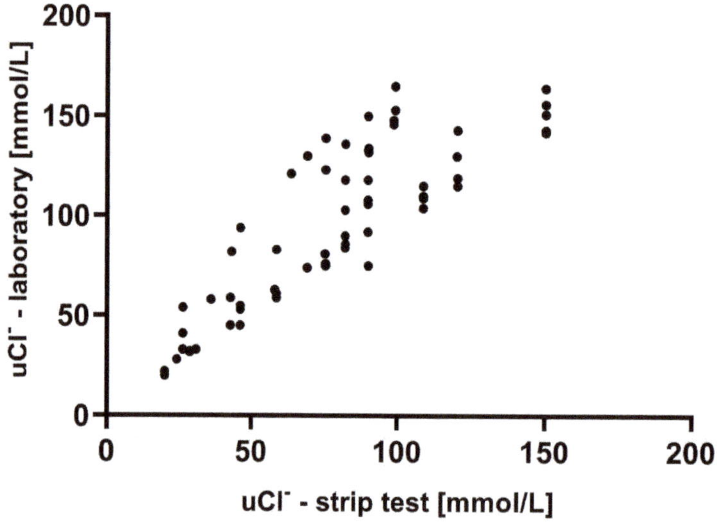

Figure 2. Relationship between urine chloride measured in the laboratory and in strip test across the entire cohort.

This equation was as follows:

$$(uCl\text{-lab}) = 1 \times (uCl\text{-strip}) + 17.94; p < 0.001 \quad (3)$$

3.3.1. The Relationship Between Urine Chloride Measured in the Laboratory and the Strip Test in HF vs. No-HF Patients

In terms of the accuracy of the uCl^- measured in the strip test (*uCl*-strip) and the uCl^- or uNa^+ evaluated in a local laboratory (*uCl*-lab and uNa-lab, respectively), the individuals with HF presented a stronger correlation between the urine chloride obtained in the strip test and in the laboratory (r = 0.88 in chronic HF and r = 0.71 in no-HF patients, $p < 0.001$ for both). The linear regression models were as follows: (*uCl*-lab) = 0.98 × (*uCl*-strip) + 15.77 ($p < 0.001$) in HF patients and (*uCl*-lab) = 0.77 × (*uCl*-strip) + 47.91 ($p < 0.001$) in no-HF individuals. This relationships are presented in Figure 3A. The subgroups' characteristics and the accuracy of fit between the laboratory and strip-established ion concentrations are presented in the Supplementary Materials.

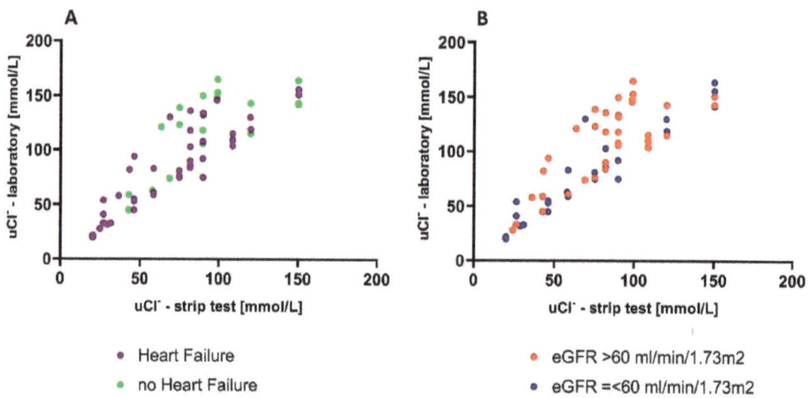

Figure 3. The relationship between urine chloride measured in the laboratory and in strip test in patients with HF vs. without HF (**A**) and with low vs. high eGFR (**B**).

3.3.2. The Relationship Between Urine Chloride Measured in the Laboratory and in the Strip Test in Low-e-GFR vs. High-eGFR Patients

We divided the whole study cohort according to eGFR (eGFR > 60 mL/min/m^2 (named: "low eGFR") and eGFR $\leq$ 60 mL/min/m^2 ("high eGFR")). A well-fitted linear pattern was observed for patients with low eGFR (N = 26) (r = 0.94, $p < 0.001$), with a linear regression equation as follows: ((*uCl*-lab) = 0.96 × (*uCl*-strip) + 11.22; $p < 0.001$). Those with high eGFR (N = 40) also presented a linear correlation between the values obtained in both tests (r = 0.74; $p < 0.001$), but this was weaker than for the low-e-GFR group. The linear regression equation was as follows: (*uCl*-lab) = 0.92 × (*uCl*-strip) + 28.20; $p < 0.001$). This relationship is presented graphically in Figure 3B. The characteristics of the subgroups and the accuracy of fit between the ion concentrations measured in the laboratory and those established by strip testing, shown on Bland–Altman plots, are provided in the Supplementary Materials.

3.4. The Relationship Between Urine Sodium Measured in the Laboratory and Urine Chloride in Strip Tests

The pattern of the relationship between uNa$^+$ laboratory measurements and uCl^- from the strip tests was weaker than in the case of urine chloride (r = 0.71; $p < 0.001$), with the following regression equation: (uNa-lab)= 0.81 × (*uCl*-strip) + 30.11; $p < 0.001$ (Figure 4).

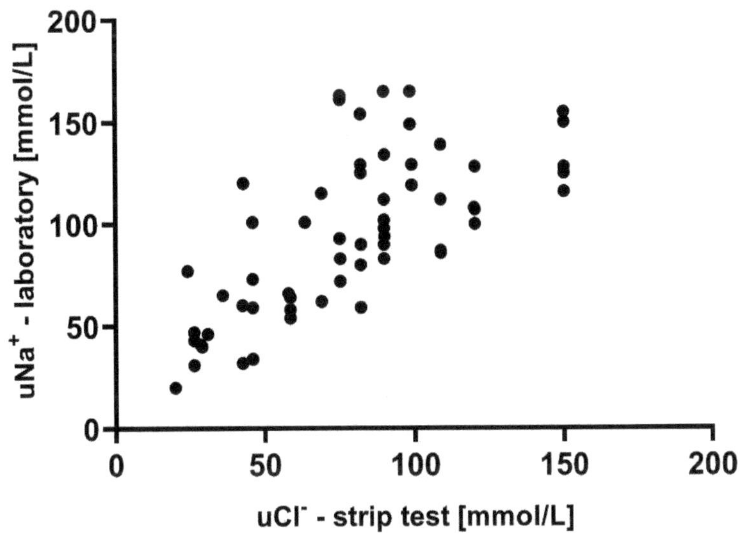

Figure 4. The relationship between urine sodium concentration measured in the laboratory and urine chloride obtained in strip tests for the entire cohort.

The correlation between both measured values in HF patients was r = 0.71 ($p < 0.001$), and in the no-HF subgroup r = 0.52 ($p = 0.02$). These linear relationships can be described by the following equations: (uNa-lab) = 0.80 × (*uCl*-strip) + 30.68; $p < 0.001$ and (uNa-lab) = 0.59 × (*uCl*-strip) + 56.16; $p = 0.02$), respectively. This is presented in Figure 5A.

The correlation between uNa-lab and *uCl*-strip was stronger for those with low eGFR (r = 0.91; $p < 0.001$) than for high eGFR (r = 0.49, $p < 0.01$), as described by the following equations: (uNa-lab) = 0.85 × (*uCl*-strip) + 16.94 ($p < 0.001$) and (uNa-lab) = 0.65 × (*uCl*-strip) + 49.93 ($p < 0.001$), respectively. The patterns of these relationships are presented in Figure 5B.

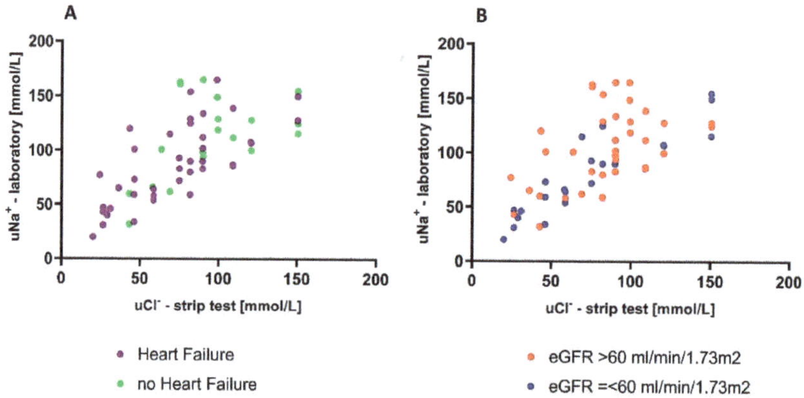

Figure 5. The relationship between urine sodium concentration measured in laboratory and urine chloride obtained in strip test in patients with HF vs. without HF (**A**) and low vs. high eGFR (**B**).

3.5. Graphical Presentation of Agreement Between Urine Chloride and Sodium Measured in Laboratory and Urine Chloride Measured in Strip Tests

The degree of agreement between urine chloride concentration obtained in strip-test and urine chloride and sodium obtained in the laboratory (gold standard) method were presented in Bland-Altmann plots (Figures 6 and 7). The subgroups analyses were presented in Supplementary Materials.

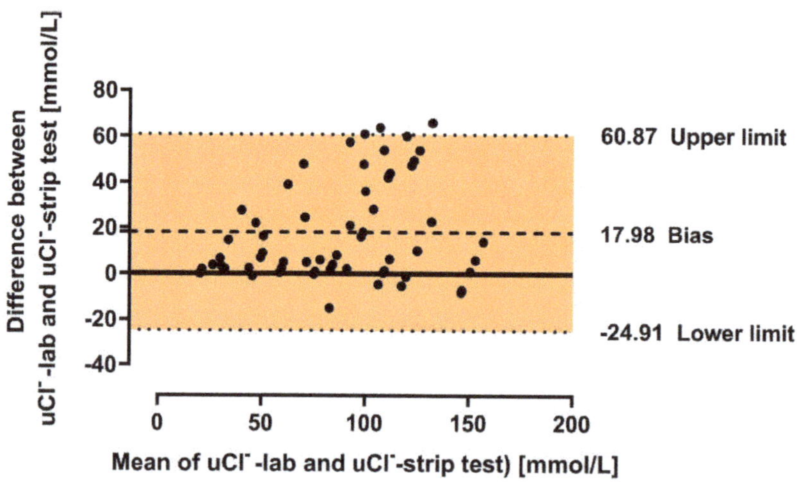

Figure 6. Bland–Altman plot for agreement of urine chloride concentration measured by strip tests and urine chloride measured in the laboratory in the general cohort. Legend: *uCl*$^-$—urine chloride; Bias—mean difference between strip test and laboratory test results; Lower limit—mean difference-1.96 × standard deviation; Upper limit—mean difference + 1.96 × standard deviation.

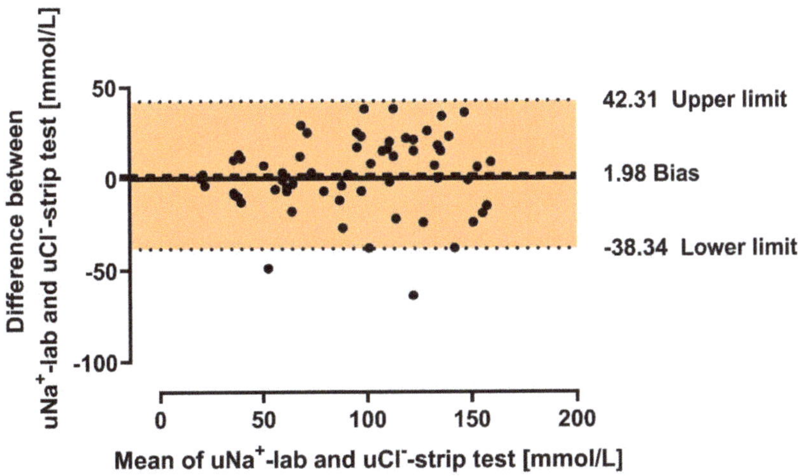

Figure 7. Bland–Altman plot for agreement of urine chloride concentration measured by strip test and urine sodium measured in the laboratory in the general cohort. Legend: uCl^{-}—urine chloride; uNa^{+}—urine sodium; Bias—mean difference between strip test and laboratory test results; Lower limit—mean difference-1.96 × standard deviation; Upper limit—mean difference + 1.96 × standard deviation.

3.6. Sensitivity, Specificity, and Positive and Negative Predictive Values of uCl^{-} Strip Test for an Indication of Poor Diuretic Response

In chronic heart failure, there is no widely established cut-off point for uNa^{+} and/or uCl^{-} indicating a poor treatment response. However, we conducted a simulation assuming a cut-off point of 70 mmol/L for both uNa^{+} and uCl^{-}, established in patients with acute heart failure, to define poor diuretic response (<70 mmol/L). We then calculated the parameters (sensitivity, specificity, and positive and negative predictive values) for the uCl^{-} strip test (<70 mmol/L) for the indication of poor treatment response, predefined using the above the cut-off point. The obtained sensitivity, specificity, and positive and negative predictive values were satisfactory (Table 2).

Table 2. Parameters of uCl^{-} strip indication for poor treatment response (cut-offs: uNa-lab < 70 mmol/L and *uCl*-strip < 70 mmol/L).

Parameter	Sensitivity	Specificity	Positive Predictive Value	Negative Predictive Value
uNa-lab < 70 mmol/L	94.7%	85.7%	75.0%	97.3%
uCl-lab < 70 mmol/L	100%	86.0%	75.0%	100%

3.7. Test Power Analysis

Based on the obtained correlation coefficients and cohort sizes, and assuming an alpha level of 0.05, the test power was approximately 1.0 for the entire study cohort when divided into the above subgroups. However, in the analysis of *uCl*-strip and uNa-lab in the non-heart failure population, the test power was 0.73.

3.8. Issues of Measurement and Notation Bias

Despite the validated method of chloride evaluation via strip test, which has been known for many years, some issues were found during the study processing. The first was the inconsistency in the pattern of the top borders of the concentration indicators across measurements. For instance, instead of a flat line, in some cases a triangle shape is seen with no clearly visible tip (Figure 8D–F). This may cause the bias of underestimation or overestimation (depending on the user assessment). For comparison, the well-visible markers were shown in Figure 8B,C. Other tests do not have sharply defined borders, but instead, their color gradually changes. An additional issue is the different times taken for patients to fill the strip and show the proper results. There were some technical issues in some cases; for some patients, the tests did not reach the marker indicating the end of the assessment (despite a long waiting time), which did not allow us to classify these tests as reliable.

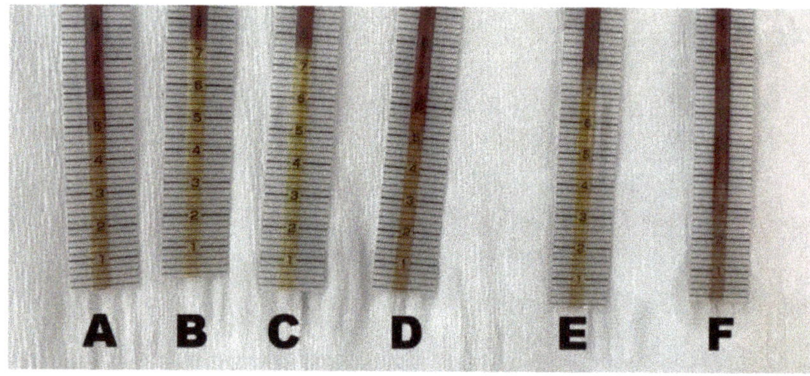

Figure 8. Examples of different patterns of urine chloride markers in the strips ((**A**)–(**F**)).

4. Discussion

The presented study shows a high correlation between the urine chloride evaluated in strip tests and urine chloride and/or sodium assessment using the gold-standard laboratory method. The results of this study reveal several significant implications.

The first one is the fact that the concentration of uCl^- was underestimated by the measurement achieved via the strip tests in comparison to the laboratory assessments. This was confirmed by the mathematical analysis of the relationship between the variables. Note that the values of *uCl*-lab are higher than *uCl*-strip for the entire population and subsequent subgroups (see equations and plots in results). Furthermore, the pattern of changes between uCl^- or uNa^+ from the laboratory tests and uCl^- obtained in the strip tests was flatter for those without HF or with high eGFR. Only in the case of urine chloride comparison regarding eGFR were the patterns of the relationship almost parallel. This raises some doubt as to whether using such tests in outpatient care in the general population as the sole marker influencing decisions regarding a possible increase in doses of diuretics might lead to overdiagnosis by the patient of conditions threatening the decompensation of chronic heart failure.

A few studies conducted using strip tests for chloride assessment have shown different degrees of correlation between the test results and laboratory measurements. These results differ between studies, showing the highest agreement in healthy individuals and slightly lower agreement in populations of patients with intestinal and neurological disorders (suspected cerebral salt-wasting). Nonetheless, there are no studies providing insight into the usefulness of chloride strip tests in heart failure [22,23]. Heart failure patients take diuretics and other drugs that chronically influence neurohormonal activity, which is overactivated in this condition. Consequently, kidney function and diuretic response are affected by these factors, leading to significant differences among heart failure patients and other tested populations [14,24–28].

Another issue is the significantly better fit of the values measured by the strip test with those obtained in laboratory assessments in patients with low eGFR compared to patients with high eGFR values. The results indicate that the model based on these values explains approximately 90% of the obtained measurements. This gives us basis to suspect that the use of strip tests in certain groups (e.g., patients with low eGFR) could be successfully applied in outpatient management, indicating the high reliability of the measurements made by educated, aware patients.

Thirdly, the chloride concentration measured using the strip test showed that there is also a significant relationship with the sodium concentration in urine (assessed in the laboratory). This relationship was inherently weaker than that for chlorides, but also showed a profile similar to the relationship between the chloride concentrations from the strip test and the laboratory measurements. Again, a significantly stronger relationship was observed in the groups of patients with HF and low eGFR. Studies have demonstrated the significant relationships of chloride established in strip tests in relation to natriuresis. Their results are similar to those obtained in our study cohort despite the different populations included in the analysis [23]. It is noteworthy that the subsequent analyses that were conducted were characterized by satisfactory test power.

Another, fourth, important topic is the various issues that may affect measurement bias, consequently impacting the checked/indicated value of the test. Note that the higher the value indicated in the strip test (on an interval scale), the greater the risk of measurement error due to the exponential relationship between this value and its assigned concentration. Hence, the lower the chloride concentration, the lesser the potential impact of measurement error on the obtained value (and potential further clinical decisions). For example, the difference between a strip test result of 4.6 and 4.8 translates to a difference in chloride concentration of 29 to 31 mmol/L, while between a reading of 8.6 and 8.8, the increase in chloride concentration is significantly greater—150 to 169 mmol/L! This is reflected in the Bland–Altman plots, where the difference between the values obtained from the strip tests and the laboratory tests increases with higher mean test values (Figures 6 and 7, and Supplementary Materials). Additionally, the issue with indicator boundaries (e.g., poor visibility or results falling between two indicator lines), as discussed in a separate section, may contribute to measurement imprecision, especially at increasing strip test values. In the study, we deliberately decided that a single investigator would read the tests to simulate the situation where a patient would need to interpret the test result during self-assessment. A consensus evaluation by multiple researchers was not conducted, as this could potentially fail to reflect the bias associated with individual assessment. An action that could be useful in the future, limiting human factors' impact on obtaining strip test results, could be the use of devices utilizing the digital analysis of ion concentrations in urine. Unfortunately, these devices are relatively more expensive and thus less accessible to patients. Additionally, no studies have proven the superiority of digital chloride/sodium assessment in urine compared to strip tests in either the heart failure population or other groups. Nevertheless, the dynamic development of digital technologies (especially artificial intelligence) may provide a tool in the future for the low-cost, simple-in-use, and reliable evaluation of biochemical body fluids. It should be highlighted that similar strip tests have been tested in the context of predicting 24 h urinary sodium excretion based on various protocols for collecting and assessing single urine samples. In these studies, flame photometry, among other methods, was used to assess sodium concentration as a reference method. The results were consistent with the strip test results [29]. Additionally, various strip tests have also been examined for their agreement with reference results, showing general consistency in three out of four tested systems, although each had its own problems—difficulty in reading the result, the need to dilute urine samples due to exceeding the test range, etc. [30].

Taking into account the presented results and discussion, the clinical applicability of this study lies in the potential use of strip tests for outpatient self-monitoring, or as a point-of-care tool for inpatients. This could become an integral element in the development of remote monitoring for patients with heart failure. In the future, such measurements could play a crucial role in home diuretic titration, which is particularly important given the association between higher doses of loop diuretics and worsening outcomes [13,31,32].

5. Conclusions

Our study shows that strip tests appear to be a highly accurate tool for uCl^- assessment, with a high correlation with the gold standard (laboratory assessment). There was a relationship between gold-standard laboratory urine chloride, sodium, and strip test chloride measurements. Nevertheless, the results were not perfectly matched. Moreover, promising data obtained in patients with low eGFR indicate the potential usefulness of chloride strip tests, with high reliability in specific populations with chronic heart failure. However, due to the limitations (relatively low sample size) and character (single-center study) of our work, multicenter, randomized studies based on sequential spot urine chloride and/or sodium assessments are necessary to extrapolate the abovementioned results onto the broad heart failure population. Additionally, dynamic developments in computer-based assessments (e.g., artificial intelligence) may be useful in the future to check strip test results.

6. Limitations

This is a single-center, observational study conducted on a relatively small population (but large enough to obtain significant testing power). This limits the generalization of the results and does not allow us to present causality. Moreover, there are no widely established urine monitoring tools to compare with the strip test in a cohort of heart failure patients.

The strip test results were assessed by a single dedicated physician, which could introduce reading bias (especially due to different patterns of result indications—see "Issues of measurement and notation bias"). Moreover, the ion concentration agreement between the strip tests and the laboratory "gold standard" was based on a single assessment. Multiple measurements using average results could potentially provide greater consistency between tests. The study design, however, deliberately promoted single-user reading to simulate the real-life scenario in which the patient would read the strip test by themself (not knowing how far individual results deviate from the actual value). However, as mentioned above, this design is related to some limitations. In clinical practice, some risk of measurement error (and variation) would be acceptable if it did not significantly affect the decision-making process. As we did not store the urine samples or strip tests during the study, we cannot compare them further with different utilities or re-assess the strip tests using multiple investigators.

Supplementary Materials: The following supporting information can be downloaded at: https://www.mdpi.com/article/10.3390/biomedicines12112473/s1.

Author Contributions: Conceptualization, P.P., M.G. and J.B.; methodology, M.G.; formal analysis, M.G.; investigation, M.G. and B.J.; data curation, M.G. and B.J.; writing—original draft preparation, M.G. and B.J.; writing—review and editing, M.G. and J.B.; visualization, M.G. and B.J.; supervision, P.P. and J.B.; project administration, M.G. All authors have read and agreed to the published version of the manuscript.

Funding: This research was financially supported by Wroclaw Medical University, Poland.

Institutional Review Board Statement: No. 229/2024, Wroclaw Medical University Ethical Committee.

Informed Consent Statement: Informed consent was obtained from all subjects involved in the study.

Data Availability Statement: Data can be shared upon explicit request.

Conflicts of Interest: P.P. reports personal fees from Boehringer Ingelheim, AstraZeneca, Servier, Bristol Myers Squibb, Amgen, Novartis, Merck, Pfizer, and Berlin Chemie, and grants and personal fees from Vifor Pharma. M.G., B.J., and J.B. have no competing interests.

References

1. Riccardi, M.; Sammartino, A.M.; Piepoli, M.; Adamo, M.; Pagnesi, M.; Rosano, G.; Metra, M.; von Haehling, S.; Tomasoni, D. Heart Failure: An Update from the Last Years and a Look at the near Future. *ESC Heart Fail.* **2022**, *9*, 3667–3693. [CrossRef] [PubMed]
2. Stevenson, L.W.; Ross, H.J.; Rathman, L.D.; Boehmer, J.P. Remote Monitoring for Heart Failure Management at Home. *J. Am. Coll. Cardiol.* **2023**, *81*, 2272–2291. [CrossRef] [PubMed]
3. Mullens, W.; Damman, K.; Harjola, V.-P.; Mebazaa, A.; Brunner-La Rocca, H.-P.; Martens, P.; Testani, J.M.; Tang, W.H.W.; Orso, F.; Rossignol, P.; et al. The Use of Diuretics in Heart Failure with Congestion—A Position Statement from the Heart Failure Association of the European Society of Cardiology. *Eur. J. Heart Fail.* **2019**, *21*, 137–155. [CrossRef]
4. McDonagh, T.A.; Metra, M.; Adamo, M.; Gardner, R.S.; Baumbach, A.; Böhm, M.; Burri, H.; Butler, J.; Celutkiene, J.; Chioncel, O.; et al. 2021 ESC Guidelines for the Diagnosis and Treatment of Acute and Chronic Heart Failure. *Eur. Heart J.* **2021**, *42*, 3599–3726. [CrossRef] [PubMed]
5. Tomasoni, D.; Vishram-Nielsen, J.K.K.; Pagnesi, M.; Adamo, M.; Lombardi, C.M.; Gustafsson, F.; Metra, M. Advanced Heart Failure: Guideline-directed Medical Therapy, Diuretics, Inotropes, and Palliative Care. *ESC Heart Fail.* **2022**, *9*, 1507–1523. [CrossRef]
6. Guzik, M.; Iwanek, G.; Fudim, M.; Zymliński, R.; Marciniak, D.; Ponikowski, P.; Biegus, J. Spot Urine Sodium as a Marker of Urine Dilution and Decongestive Abilities in Acute Heart Failure. *Sci. Rep.* **2024**, *14*, 1494. [CrossRef]
7. Biegus, J.; Zymliński, R.; Testani, J.; Marciniak, D.; Zdanowicz, A.; Jankowska, E.A.; Banasiak, W.; Ponikowski, P. Renal Profiling Based on Estimated Glomerular Filtration Rate and Spot Urine Sodium Identifies High-risk Acute Heart Failure Patients. *Eur. J. Heart Fail.* **2021**, *23*, 729–739. [CrossRef]
8. Dauw, J.; Charaya, K.; Lelonek, M.; Zegri-Reiriz, I.; Nasr, S.; Paredes-Paucar, C.P.; Borbély, A.; Erdal, F.; Benkouar, R.; Cobo-Marcos, M.; et al. Protocolized Natriuresis-Guided Decongestion Improves Diuretic Response: The Multicenter ENACT-HF Study. *Circ. Heart Fail.* **2024**, *17*, e011105. [CrossRef]
9. ter Maaten, J.M.; Beldhuis, I.E.; van der Meer, P.; Krikken, J.A.; Postmus, D.; Coster, J.E.; Nieuwland, W.; van Veldhuisen, D.J.; Voors, A.A.; Damman, K. Natriuresis-Guided Diuretic Therapy in Acute Heart Failure: A Pragmatic Randomized Trial. *Nat. Med.* **2023**, *29*, 2625–2632. [CrossRef]
10. Jung, S.; Bosch, A.; Kolwelter, J.; Striepe, K.; Kannenkeril, D.; Schuster, T.; Ott, C.; Achenbach, S.; Schmieder, R.E. Renal and Intraglomerular Haemodynamics in Chronic Heart Failure with Preserved and Reduced Ejection Fraction. *ESC Heart Fail.* **2021**, *8*, 1562–1570. [CrossRef]
11. Kataoka, H. Chloride in Heart Failure Syndrome: Its Pathophysiologic Role and Therapeutic Implication. *Cardiol. Ther.* **2021**, *10*, 407–428. [CrossRef] [PubMed]
12. Kataoka, H. Mechanistic Insights into Chloride-related Heart Failure Progression According to the Plasma Volume Status. *ESC Heart Fail.* **2022**, *9*, 2044–2048. [CrossRef] [PubMed]
13. Seko, Y.; Kato, T.; Morimoto, T.; Yaku, H.; Inuzuka, Y.; Tamaki, Y.; Ozasa, N.; Shiba, M.; Yamamoto, E.; Yoshikawa, Y.; et al. Association between Changes in Loop Diuretic Dose and Outcomes in Acute Heart Failure. *ESC Heart Fail.* **2023**, *10*, 1757–1770. [CrossRef] [PubMed]
14. Matsumoto, S.; Nakamura, N.; Konishi, M.; Shibata, A.; Kida, K.; Ishii, S.; Ikeda, T.; Ikari, Y. Neuroendocrine Hormone Status and Diuretic Response to Atrial Natriuretic Peptide in Patients with Acute Heart Failure. *ESC Heart Fail.* **2022**, *9*, 4077–4087. [CrossRef]
15. Fonarow, G.C.; Adams, K.F.; Abraham, W.T.; Yancy, C.W.; Boscardin, W.J.; ADHERE Scientific Advisory Committee. Risk Stratification for In-Hospital Mortality in Acutely Decompensated Heart Failure: Classification and Regression Tree Analysis. *JAMA* **2005**, *293*, 572. [CrossRef]
16. Llàcer, P.; Croset, F.; Núñez, J.; Campos, J.; Fernández, C.; Fabregate, M.; Del Hoyo, B.; Ruiz, R.; López, G.; Tello, S.; et al. Prognostic Significance of Plasma Chloride in Elderly Patients Hospitalized for Acute Heart Failure. *ESC Heart Fail.* **2023**, *10*, 2637–2647. [CrossRef]
17. Seo, M.; Watanabe, T.; Yamada, T.; Yano, M.; Hayashi, T.; Nakagawa, A.; Nakagawa, Y.; Tamaki, S.; Yasumura, Y.; Sotomi, Y.; et al. Prognostic Significance of Serum Chloride Level in Heart Failure Patients with Preserved Ejection Fraction. *ESC Heart Fail.* **2022**, *9*, 1444–1453. [CrossRef]
18. Van den Eynde, J.; Verbrugge, F.H. Renal Sodium Avidity in Heart Failure. *Cardiorenal. Med.* **2024**, *14*, 270–280. [CrossRef]
19. Kono, H.; Kitai, T.; Kim, K.; Kobori, A.; Ehara, N.; Kinoshita, M.; Kaji, S.; Furukawa, Y. Fractional Excretion of Sodium after the Treatment of Acute Decompensated Heart Failure Predicts the Prognosis. *J. Am. Coll. Cardiol.* **2019**, *73*, 1002. [CrossRef]
20. Watanabe, Y.; Kubota, Y.; Nishino, T.; Tara, S.; Kato, K.; Hayashi, D.; Mozawa, K.; Matsuda, J.; Tokita, Y.; Yasutake, M.; et al. Utility of Fractional Excretion of Urea Nitrogen in Heart Failure Patients with Chronic Kidney Disease. *ESC Heart Fail.* **2023**, *10*, 1706–1716. [CrossRef]
21. van der Wal, M.H.L.; Jaarsma, T.; Jenneboer, L.C.; Linssen, G.C.M. Thirst in Stable Heart Failure Patients; Time to Reconsider Fluid Restriction and Prescribed Diuretics. *ESC Heart Fail.* **2022**, *9*, 2181–2188. [CrossRef] [PubMed]
22. Jeffery, R.W.; Mullenbach, V.A.; Bjornson-Benson, W.M.; Prineas, R.J.; Forster, J.L.; Schlundt, D.G. Home Testing of Urine Chloride to Estimate Dietary Sodium Intake: Evaluation of Feasibility and Accuracy. *Addict. Behav.* **1987**, *12*, 17–21. [CrossRef] [PubMed]

23. Hamilton, F.W.; Penfold, C.M.; Ness, A.R.; Stevenson, K.P.; Atkinson, C.; Day, A.M.; Sebepos-Rogers, G.M.; Tyrrell-Price, J. Can Quantab Titrator Sticks Reliably Predict Urinary Sodium? *Clin. Nutr. ESPEN* **2018**, *23*, 217–221. [CrossRef] [PubMed]
24. Kaissling, B.; Bachmann, S.; Kriz, W. Structural Adaptation of the Distal Convoluted Tubule to Prolonged Furosemide Treatment. *Am. J. Physiol.-Ren. Physiol.* **1985**, *248*, F374–F381. [CrossRef] [PubMed]
25. Biegus, J.; Zymliński, R.; Testani, J.; Fudim, M.; Cox, Z.L.; Guzik, M.; Iwanek, G.; Hurkacz, M.; Raj, D.; Marciniak, D.; et al. The Blunted Loop Diuretic Response in Acute Heart Failure Is Driven by Reduced Tubular Responsiveness Rather than Insufficient Tubular Delivery. The Role of Furosemide Urine Excretion on Diuretic and Natriuretic Response in Acute Heart Failure. *Eur. J. Heart Fail.* **2023**, *25*, 1323–1333. [CrossRef]
26. Biegus, J.; Mebazaa, A.; Davison, B.; Cotter, G.; Edwards, C.; Čelutkienė, J.; Chioncel, O.; Cohen-Solal, A.; Filippatos, G.; Novosadova, M.; et al. Effects of Rapid Uptitration of Neurohormonal Blockade on Effective, Sustainable Decongestion and Outcomes in STRONG-HF. *J. Am. Coll. Cardiol.* **2024**, *84*, 323–336. [CrossRef]
27. Mebazaa, A.; Davison, B.A.; Biegus, J.; Edwards, C.; Murtagh, G.; Varounis, C.; Hayrapetyan, H.; Sisakian, H.; Ter-Grigoryan, V.R.; Takagi, K.; et al. Reduced Congestion and Improved Response to a Fluid/Sodium Challenge in Chronic Heart Failure Patients after Initiation of Sacubitril/Valsartan: The NATRIUM-HF study. *Eur. J. Heart Fail.* **2024**, *26*, 1507–1517. [CrossRef]
28. Biegus, J.; Nawrocka-Millward, S.; Zymliński, R.; Fudim, M.; Testani, J.; Marciniak, D.; Rosiek-Biegus, M.; Ponikowska, B.; Guzik, M.; Garus, M.; et al. Distinct Renin/Aldosterone Activity Profiles Correlate with Renal Function, Natriuretic Response, Decongestive Ability and Prognosis in Acute Heart Failure. *Int. J. Cardiol.* **2021**, *345*, 54–60. [CrossRef]
29. Heeney, N.D.; Lee, R.H.; Hockin, B.C.D.; Clarke, D.C.; Sanatani, S.; Armstrong, K.; Sedlak, T.; Claydon, V.E. At-Home Determination of 24-h Urine Sodium Excretion: Validation of Chloride Test Strips and Multiple Spot Samples. *Auton. Neurosci.* **2021**, *233*, 102797. [CrossRef]
30. Brüngel, M.; Kluthe, R.; Fürst, P. Evaluation of Various Rapid Chloride Tests for Assessing Urinary NaCl Excretion. *Ann. Nutr. Metab.* **2001**, *45*, 169–174. [CrossRef]
31. Baudry, G.; Coutance, G.; Dorent, R.; Bauer, F.; Blanchart, K.; Boignard, A.; Chabanne, C.; Delmas, C.; D'Ostrevy, N.; Epailly, E.; et al. Diuretic Dose Is a Strong Prognostic Factor in Ambulatory Patients Awaiting Heart Transplantation. *ESC Heart Fail.* **2023**, *10*, 2843–2852. [CrossRef] [PubMed]
32. Eshaghian, S.; Horwich, T.B.; Fonarow, G.C. Relation of Loop Diuretic Dose to Mortality in Advanced Heart Failure. *Am. J. Cardiol.* **2006**, *97*, 1759–1764. [CrossRef] [PubMed]

biomedicines

MDPI

Article

Insights into the Associations Between Systolic Left Ventricular Rotational Mechanics and Left Atrial Peak Reservoir Strains in Healthy Adults from the MAGYAR-Healthy Study

Attila Nemes *, Árpád Kormányos, Nóra Ambrus and Csaba Lengyel

Department of Medicine, Albert Szent-Györgyi Medical School, University of Szeged, Semmelweis Street 8, P.O. Box 427, H-6725 Szeged, Hungary; kormanyos.arpad@med.u-szeged.hu (Á.K.); ambrusnora@gmail.com (N.A.); lecs@in1st.szote.u-szeged.hu (C.L.)

* Correspondence: nemes.attila@med.u-szeged.hu; Tel.: +36-62-545220; Fax: +36-62-544568

Abstract: Introduction: In systole, when the left ventricle (LV) twists, the left atrium (LA) behaves like a reservoir, having a special wall contractility pattern opposite to that of the LV wall. Accordingly, the objective of the present study was to investigate the associations between LV rotational mechanics and LA peak (reservoir) strains as assessed simultaneously by three-dimensional speckle-tracking echocardiography (3DSTE) under healthy conditions. Methods: In the present study, 157 healthy adults (mean age: 33.2 ± 12.7 years, 73 men) were involved. Complete two-dimensional Doppler echocardiography with 3DSTE-derived data acquisition were performed in all cases. The 3DSTE-derived LV rotational and LA strain parameters were determined at a later date. Results: Global LA peak reservoir circumferential (22.7 ± 6.4% vs. 27.6 ± 6.8%, $p < 0.05$) and area (57.8 ± 20.0% vs. 66.0 ± 22.7%, $p < 0.05$) strains proved to be reduced in the case of the highest vs. lowest basal LV rotation; other LA peak reservoir strains were not associated with increasing basal LV rotation. Global LA peak radial strain was highest in the case of the lowest vs. highest apical LV rotation (−19.2 ± 9.4% vs. −13.0 ± 8.2%, $p < 0.05$). Global LA peak reservoir 3D strain was lowest in the case of the highest vs. lowest apical LV rotation (−9.9 ± 6.8% vs. −5.0 ± 4.2%, $p < 0.05$). Only apical LV rotation proved to be significantly reduced in the case of the highest vs. lowest global LA peak reservoir 3D strain (8.12 ± 3.23° vs. 10.50 ± 3.44°, $p < 0.05$). Other global LA peak reservoir strains were not associated with basal and apical LV rotations. Conclusions: In LV systole, LV rotational mechanics is associated with LA deformation represented by LA peak (reservoir) strains even in healthy circumstances. While basal LV rotation is associated with LA widening, apical LV rotation is associated with LA thinning, suggesting the close cooperation of the LV and LA in systole even in healthy adults.

Keywords: left ventricular; rotation; left atrial; strain; three-dimensional; echocardiography

1. Introduction

It is well known that the heart cycle consists of two parts: diastole and systole. In the latter, the left ventricle (LV) is emptied through the aortic valve with the mitral valve closed [1]. The movement of the LV is complex during systole, as in addition to wall contractions represented by deformation parameters [2], it twists like the wringing of a towel at the same time as well. The apical part of the LV rotates in the counterclockwise direction, and its base rotates in the clockwise direction. With this form of movement, the rate of ejection is optimized [3–7]. During LV twist or rotational mechanics, the left atrium (LA) behaves like a reservoir, and its volume is the largest. In this phase of LA function, the direction of its wall movement is opposite to that of the LV wall, and it can be quantitatively characterized using strains. In systole, thinning, widening and lengthening of LA walls in the radial, circumferential and longitudinal directions can be detected, and these changes are represented by specific so-called LA peak or reservoir strains, respectively [2,8,9]. The fact is that systolic LV rotational mechanics and simultaneous LA contractility, and the deformation parameters representing them, have not been sufficiently investigated within clinical circumstances. Three-dimensional (3D) speckle-tracking echocardiography (3DSTE) provides an easy-to-learn/easy-to-perform method with a non-invasive approach to examining the above mechanisms and creates an opportunity to perform physiological studies at the same time [10–13]. Accordingly, the objective of the present study was to examine the association between 3DSTE-derived characteristics of LV rotational mechanics and LA peak reservoir strains under healthy conditions by examining what would happen when these parameters were smaller or greater than the average as well. Whether the regional LV rotations showed a correlation with different deformation parameters representing the 3D contractility of the LA in systole was also investigated.

2. Subjects and Methods

2.1. Subject Population

In this study, 157 healthy adult individuals (mean age: 33.2 ± 12.7 years, 73 men) were involved, with LV rotational mechanics being in the normal direction being confirmed in all individuals. The enrollment of all volunteers was carried out between 2011 and 2017. In all cases, laboratory testing, physical examination, standard 12-lead electrocardiography (ECG) and two-dimensional (2D) Doppler echocardiography were performed with negative results. No one used any medications or was a smoker, professional athlete or obese. If someone had a disease or clinical condition that could have affected the results, they were excluded from the study. The 3DSTE-based data acquisition was conducted at the same time as 2D Doppler echocardiography in accordance with the latest guidelines and practices. The detailed 3DSTE-based analysis was carried out offline at a later date [1–4]. The present retrospective study is part of the 'Motion Analysis of the heart and Great vessels bY three-dimensionAl speckle-tRacking echocardiography in Healthy subjects' study (MAGYAR-Healthy Study), which was organized partly to perform physiological analyses between 3DSTE-derived parameters in healthy adults ('Magyar' means 'Hungarian' in the Hungarian language). This study was conducted in accordance with the Declaration of Helsinki (as revised in 2013). All participants gave informed consent and the Institutional and Regional Human Biomedical Research Committee of the University of Szeged, Hungary (No.: 71/2011), approved this study.

2.2. Two-Dimensional Doppler Echocardiography

The Toshiba Artida™ echocardiography tool was used on all individuals (Toshiba Medical Systems, Tokyo, Japan), attached to a PST-30BT (1–5 MHz) phased-array transducer for a complete analysis. Complete routine 2D echocardiographic assessment of heart chambers and valves was conducted in all healthy individuals. Studies included the quantification of the LA and LV, exclusion of significant valve stenoses and regurgitations by Doppler echocardiography, and pulsed Doppler assessment of early (E) and late (A) diastolic mitral inflow velocities and their ratios (E/A) [1].

2.3. Three-Dimensional Speckle-Tracking Echocardiography

The same Toshiba Artida™ cardiac ultrasound device attached to a PST-25SX matrix transducer with 3D capability was used for the 3DSTE scans. During the studies, subjects in sinus rhythm lay in the left lateral decubitus position, and then 3D echocardiographic datasets were acquired from an apical window, while the subject held his/her breath. To achieve optimal images, 6 subvolumes were acquired over 6 cardiac cycles, and the software automatically combined these subvolumes into a full-volume 3D echocardiographic dataset. Detailed data analysis was carried out offline at a later time using version 2.7 of the manufacturer's 3D Wall Motion Tracking software (Ultra Extend, Toshiba Medical Systems, Tokyo, Japan) [10–13].

2.4. Determination of LV Rotational Mechanics

To quantify the LV rotational mechanics, apical longitudinal views were selected in apical 4-chamber (AP4CH) and 2-chamber (AP2CH) views, as well as basal, midventricular and apical cross-sectional planes, and the mitral annular (MA) ring—LV edges and endocardial surface of the LV apex were determined. Then, after sequential analysis, a virtual 3D cast of the LV was created (Figure 1) [14]. According to our own practice, we defined the following features of LV rotational mechanics from the same 3D cast of the LV:

- clockwise basal LV rotation (in degrees);
- counterclockwise apical LV rotation (in degrees);
- LV twist (net difference in LV apical and basal rotations in degrees);
- time-to-peak LV twist (in milliseconds).

If the direction of the LV apical and basal rotations were the same, clockwise or counterclockwise, LV twist was absent. This phenomenon is called LV 'rigid body rotation' (RBR). Individuals with LV-RBR were excluded from the present study [14].

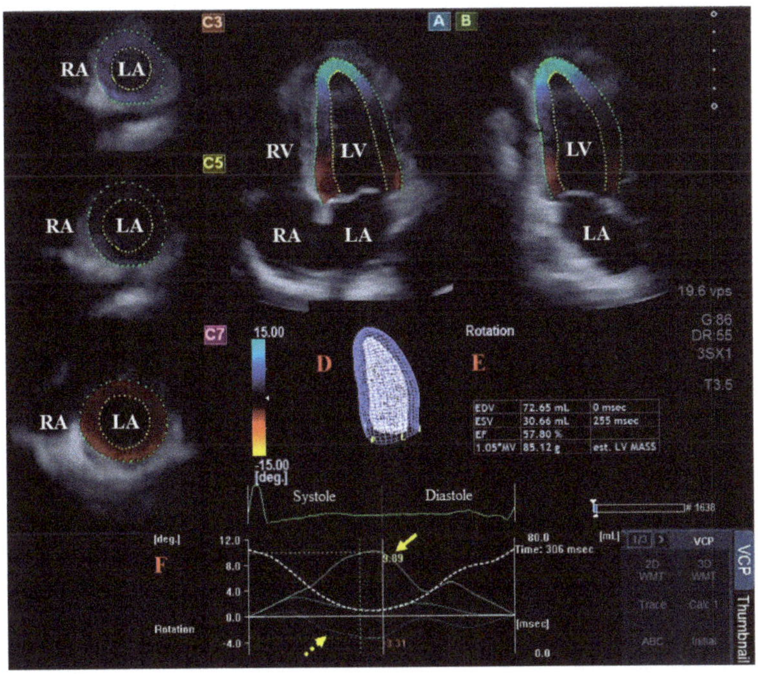

Figure 1. Three-dimensional (3D) speckle-tracking echocardiography-derived evaluation of the left ventricle (LV): apical four-chamber (**A**) and apical two-chamber long-axis views (**B**), and short-axis view at basal (**C3**), midventricular (**C5**) and apical LV levels (**C7**) are demonstrated together with a 3D cast of the LV (**D**) and calculated LV volumetric data (**E**). Apical (yellow arrow) and basal LV rotational curves (dashed yellow arrow) together with LV volume change curve during the heart cycle (dashed white curve) (**F**). Abbreviations. EDV, end-diastolic volume; EF, ejection fraction; ESV, end-systolic volume; LA, left atrium; LV, left ventricle; RA, right atrium; RV, right ventricle.

2.5. Determination of LA Strains

By using the same software, at the end of the diastole, AP4CH and AP2CH views, as well as 3 short-axis views at the apical, midatrial and superior LA levels, were automatically selected on LA-focused images. After image optimizations, the endocardial LA boundary was detected by adjusting multiple markers from the edge of the septum-MA towards the edge of the LV lateral wall-MA. Then, automatic reconstruction of the LA endocardial surface was performed, allowing strain analyses. Several global LA strains representing the whole LA were determined [2,8,9]:

2.5.1. Unidimensional/Unidirectional Global LA Strains

- Radial strain (GRS) representing thickening and thinning of the myocardial walls;
- Longitudinal strain (GLS) representing lengthening and shortening of the myocardial walls;
- Circumferential strain (GCS) representing widening and narrowing of the myocardial walls.

2.5.2. Multidimensional/Multidirectional Complex LA Strains

- Area strain (GAS) is a combination of GLS and GCS.
- 3D strain (G3DS) is a combination of GRS, GLS and GCS.

Twin-peak strain curves were detected, where the first represented reservoir function of the LA in systole, while the second represented atrial contraction at end-diastole (LA systole) (Figure 2). In the present study, systolic LA peak reservoir strains were used for analysis [2,8,9].

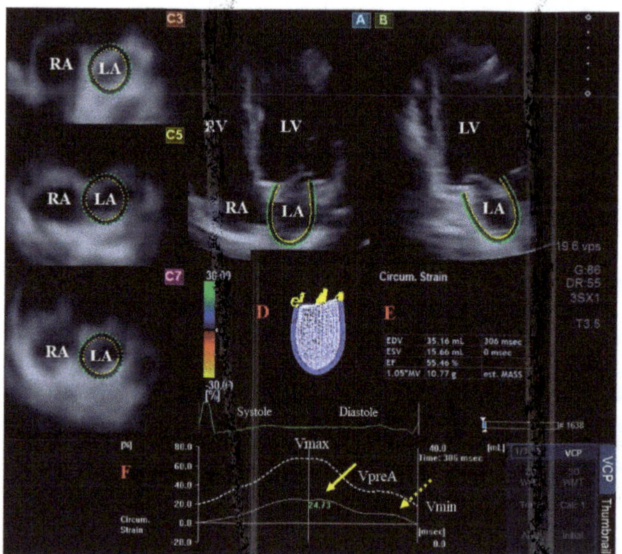

Figure 2. Three-dimensional (3D) speckle-tracking echocardiography-derived evaluation of the left atrium (LA): apical four-chamber (**A**) and two-chamber long-axis views (**B**), and short-axis view at basal (**C3**), midatrial (**C5**) and superior LA levels (**C7**) demonstrated with a 3D cast of the LA (**D**) and calculated LA volumetric data (**E**). Time—global LA volume change (dashed white curve) and time—LA global longitudinal strain change (white curve) respecting the heart cycle are demonstrated (**F**). LA peak reservoir strains and LA strains at atrial contraction are presented with yellow and dashed yellow arrows, respectively. Abbreviations. EDV, end-diastolic volume, EF, ejection fraction, ESV, end-systolic volume, LA, left atrium, LV, left ventricle, RA, right atrium, RV, right ventricle, Vmax, maximum volume of the LA, VpreA, preatrial contraction LA volume, Vmin, minimum volume of the LA.

2.6. Statistical Analysis

The mean ± standard deviation (SD) format was used for continuous variables, while the number/percent format was used for categorical variables. The difference was significant if $p < 0.05$. The normality was tested by the Shapiro–Wilk test: in the case of a normal distribution of continuous variables, Student's t-test with Welch correction was used, while when distribution was non-normal, the Mann–Whitney–Wilcoxon test was performed. Intra- and inter-observer agreements were tested by interclass correlation coefficients (ICCs). SPSS software was used during statistical analyses (SPSS Inc., version 22, Chicago, IL, USA).

3. Results

3.1. Clinical and Two-Dimensional Doppler Echocardiographic Data

From the echo data, the LA diameter was measured in the parasternal long-axis view (36.8 ± 4.0 mm) together with LV end-diastolic diameter (48.1 ± 3.7 mm) and volume (106.5 ± 22.8 mL), LV end-systolic diameter (40.8 ± 26.2 mm) and volume (36.3 ± 9.0 mL), interventricular septum (8.9 ± 1.6 mm), LV posterior wall (9.1 ± 1.7 mm), and LV ejection fraction (66.0 ± 4.9%), all were being in the normal ranges. The mean E/A proved to be 1.37 ± 0.38. Significant valvular stenosis or valvular regurgitation larger than grade 1 could not be confirmed in any valves in any cases.

3.2. Classification of Subjects

3DSTE-derived LA peak reservoir strains and parameters featuring the LV rotational mechanics of healthy individuals are demonstrated in Table 1. The group of healthy controls were classified into three subgroups according to their normal basal and apical LV rotations, peak LA-GRS, LA-GCS, LA-GLS, LA-G3DS and LA-GAS: the estimated mean ± SD served as the lower (2.18 degree, 5.95 degree, 6.73%, 18.33%, 17.43%, 1.75% and 39.63%, respectively) and larger (6.34 degree, 13.03 degree, 22.73%, 49.31%, 35.51%, 13.07% and 96.41%, respectively) values.

Table 1. Three-dimensional speckle-tracking echocardiography-derived left atrial peak reservoir strains and left ventricular rotational parameters.

Parameter	Measure
Left Atrial Volumes	
Maximum Left Atrial Volume (mL)	40.5 ± 12.8
Preatrial Contraction Left Atrial Volume (mL)	27.4 ± 11.3
Minimum Left Atrial Volume (mL)	19.1 ± 7.8
Systolic Left Atrial Peak Reservoir Strains	
Left Atrial Global Radial Strain (%)	−14.7 ± 8.0
Left Atrial Global Circumferential Strain (%)	33.8 ± 15.5
Left Atrial Global Longitudinal Strain (%)	26.5 ± 9.0
Left Atrial Global Three-Dimensional Strain (%)	−7.3 ± 5.7
Left Atrial Global Area Strain (%)	68.0 ± 28.4
Left Ventricular Volume-Based Parameters	
End-Diastolic Left Ventricular Volume (mL)	85.6 ± 23.2
Body Surface Area-Indexed End-Diastolic Left Ventricular Volume (mL/m^2)	46.5 ± 13.1
End-Systolic Left Ventricular Volume (mL)	36.1 ± 10.5
Body Surface Area-Indexed End-Systolic Left Ventricular Volume (mL/m^2)	19.6 ± 5.6
Left Ventricular Ejection Fraction (mL)	58.3 ± 5.7
Left Ventricular Mass (g)	158.1 ± 32.0
Systolic Left Ventricular Rotational Mechanics	
Basal Left Ventricular Rotation (Basal LVrot, °)	−4.26 ± 2.08
Apical Left Ventricular Rotation (Apical LVrot, °)	9.49 ± 3.54
Left Ventricular Twist (LVtwist, °)	13.75 ± 3.70
Time-to-LVtwist (ms)	344 ± 130

3.3. Increase in Basal or Apical LV Rotations

Increased basal LV rotation is associated with a decreasing tendency of rotation of the LV apex and increased LV twist. Increased rotation of the LV apex is associated with a decreasing tendency of rotation of the LV base and increased LV twist (Table 2).

Table 2. Peak left atrial strains and left ventricular rotational parameters in different basal and apical left ventricular rotations groups.

	Basal LV Rotation ≤ −2.18° (n = 17)	−2.18° < Basal LV Rotation < −6.34° (n = 116)	−6.34° ≤ Basal LV Rotation (n = 23)	Apical LV Rotation ≤ 5.95° (n = 24)	5.95° < Apical LV Rotation < 13.03° (n = 106)	13.03° < Apical LV Rotation (n = 27)
LA-GRS (%)	−13.3 ± 7.2	−14.5 ± 7.6	−16.8 ± 9.9	−19.2 ± 9.4	−14.2 ± 7.2 ‡	−13.0 ± 8.2 ‡
LA-GLS (%)	30.7 ± 13.7	35.1 ± 16.3	30.0 ± 11.8	35.2 ± 14.4	34.0 ± 15.3	31.9 ± 17.0
LA-GCS (%)	27.6 ± 6.8	27.1 ± 9.6	22.7 ± 6.4 *,†	24.0 ± 7.1	27.3 ± 9.4	25.2 ± 8.5
LA-G3DS (%)	−7.0 ± 5.1	−7.1 ± 5.4	−9.0 ± 6.9	−9.9 ± 6.8	−7.5 ± 5.5	−5.0 ± 4.2 ‡,#
LA-GAS (%)	66.0 ± 22.7	70.5 ± 20.2	57.8 ± 20.0 †	66.6 ± 23.5	69.2 ± 28.2	64.7 ± 32.6
Basal LV rotation (°)	−1.52 ± 0.50	−3.84 ± 1.07 *	−8.09 ± 1.16 *,†	−5.05 ± 2.10	−4.25 ± 2.08	−3.60 ± 1.76 ‡
Apical LV rotation (°)	10.93 ± 3.45	9.51 ± 3.50	8.37 ± 3.50 *	4.58 ± 0.97	9.11 ± 1.76 ‡	15.37 ± 1.90 ‡,#
LV twist (°)	12.5 ± 3.5	13.35 ± 3.44	16.45 ± 3.73 *,†	9.63 ± 2.27	13.36 ± 2.57 ‡	18.98 ± 2.49 ‡,#
Time-to-LV twist (ms)	276 ± 92	355 ± 140 *	339 ± 84 *	318 ± 150	349 ± 131	345 ± 106

* $p < 0.05$ vs. basal LV rotation ≤ 2.18 degree; † $p < 0.05$ vs. 2.18 degree < basal LV rotation < 6.34 degree; ‡ $p < 0.05$ vs. apical LV rotation ≤ 5.95 degree; # $p < 0.05$ vs. 5.95 degree < apical LV rotation < 13.03 degree. Abbreviations. LA, left atrial; LV, left ventricular; G3DS, global three-dimensional strain; GAS, global area strain; GCS, global circumferential strain; GLS, global longitudinal strain; GRS, global radial strain.

3.4. Increased LV Rotations and LA Peak Reservoir Strain

Peak LA-GCS and LA-GAS proved to be reduced in the case of the highest basal LV rotation, while other LA peak reservoir strains did not show an association with increasing basal LV rotation. Peak LA-GRS was highest in the case of the lowest apical LV rotation. Peak LA-3DS was lowest in the case of the highest apical LV rotation (Table 2).

3.5. Increase in LA Peak Reservoir Strains

All LA peak reservoir strains showed an increasing tendency of the other strains but to different extents. With increasing peak LA-GRS, increasing peak LA-GLS, LA-GCS and LA-GAS could be detected, but only up to a point, beyond which further increase could not be detected (except peak LA-G3DS). Increasing peak LA-GCS was associated with increase in all other strains except for peak LA-G3DS (only up to a point). An increase in all LA peak reservoir strains could be seen with increasing peak LA-GLS, except for peak LA-GRS (only up to a point). From complex strains, with increasing peak LA-G3DS, increasing peak LA-GLS, LA-GCS and LA-GAS could be detected, but only up to a point, beyond which further increases could not be detected (except peak LA-GRS). An increase in all LA peak reservoir strains could be detected with increasing peak LA-GAS, but only up to a point, beyond which further increases in LA peak reservoir strains could not be detected (Tables 3 and 4).

Table 3. Left atrial peak reservoir strains and left ventricular rotational parameters in different left atrial peak reservoir unidimensional strain groups.

	LA-GRS ≤ −6.73% (n = 22)	−6.73% < LA-GRS < −22.73% (n = 117)	−22.73% ≤ LA-GRS (n = 18)	LA-GCS ≤ 18.33% (n = 24)	18.33% < LA-GCS < 49.31% (n = 106)	49.31% ≤ LA-GCS (n = 27)	LA-GLS ≤ 17.43% (n = 23)	17.43% < LA-GLS < 35.51% (n = 110)	35.51% ≤ LA-GLS (n = 24)
LA-GRS (%)	−2.9 ± 2.3	−14.8 ± 4.6 *	−28.9 ± 6.6 *,†	−10.1 ± 7.0	−14.8 ± 7.8 ‡	−18.4 ± 7.6 ‡,#	−10.4 ± 8.6	−15.5 ± 8.1 $	−15.4 ± 5.4 $
LA-GLS (%)	24.2 ± 10.8	34.9 ± 15.4 *	38.2 ± 16.5 *	13.5 ± 3.6	31.9 ± 7.9 ‡	59.4 ± 10.5 ‡,#	22.2 ± 12.2	34.5 ± 15.2 $	41.9 ± 12.9 $,&
LA-GCS (%)	20.0 ± 8.4	27.7 ± 8.8 *	26.1 ± 8.1 *	18.1 ± 5.4	26.9 ± 8.2 ‡	32.2 ± 9.6 ‡,#	13.5 ± 3.4	26.0 ± 4.9 $	41.3 ± 6.0 $,&
LA-G3DS (%)	−0.8 ± 1.1	−7.6 ± 4.3 *	−14.1 ± 7.8 *,†	−4.6 ± 4.0	−7.9 ± 6.1 ‡	−7.9 ± 4.1 ‡	−4.9 ± 5.6	−7.5 ± 5.8 $	−9.2 ± 4.4 $
LA-GAS (%)	48.9 ± 25.5	71.2 ± 27.0 *	70.4 ± 31.2 *	31.7 ± 8.4	65.6 ± 18.2 ‡	110.0 ± 19.8 ‡,#	35.6 ± 17.2	68.2 ± 23.9 $	98.3 ± 21.6 $,&
Basal LV rotation (°)	−4.29 ± 1.66	−4.18 ± 2.09	−4.75 ± 2.37	−4.09 ± 1.87	−4.33 ± 2.18	−4.13 ± 1.77	−4.32 ± 2.14	−4.32 ± 2.15	−3.94 ± 1.56
Apical LV rotation (°)	9.54 ± 2.92	9.56 ± 3.64	9.00 ± 3.51	10.46 ± 3.78	9.18 ± 3.43	9.86 ± 3.55	9.67 ± 4.26	9.47 ± 3.48	9.45 ± 3.01
LV twist (°)	13.83 ± 3.00	13.74 ± 3.72	13.75 ± 4.28	14.55 ± 3.46	13.52 ± 3.72	13.99 ± 3.68	13.99 ± 4.04	13.78 ± 3.77	13.39 ± 2.86
Time-to-LV twist (ms)	339 ± 109	340 ± 116	374 ± 210	346 ± 91	351 ± 144	312 ± 95	342 ± 116	338 ± 127	368 ± 151

* $p < 0.05$ vs. LA-GRS ≤ −6.73%; † $p < 0.05$ vs. −6.73% < LA-GRS < −22.73%; ‡ $p < 0.05$ vs. LA-GCS ≤ 18.33%; # $p < 0.05$ vs. 18.33% < LA-GCS < 49.31%; $ $p < 0.05$ vs. LA-GLS ≤ 17.43%; & $p < 0.05$ vs. 17.43% < LA-GLS < 35.51%. Abbreviations. LA, left atrial; LV, left ventricular; G3DS, global three-dimensional strain; GAS, global area strain; GCS, global circumferential strain; GLS, global longitudinal strain; GRS, global radial strain.

Table 4. Left atrial peak reservoir strains and left ventricular rotational parameters in different left atrial peak reservoir complex strain groups.

	LA-G3DS ≤ 1.75% (n = 27)	1.75% < LA-G3DS < 13.07% (n = 107)	13.07% ≤ LA-G3DS (n = 23)	LA-GAS ≤ 39.63% (n = 27)	39.63% < LA-GAS < 96.41% (n = 106)	96.41% ≤ LA-GAS (n = 24)
LA-GRS (%)	−6.8 ± 7.4	−14.8 ± 5.5 *	−24.0 ± 8.6 *,†	−10.4 ± 7.7	−15.2 ± 7.9 ‡	−17.6 ± 6.8 ‡
LA-GLS (%)	26.7 ± 12.8	35.6 ± 15.9 *	34.0 ± 13.8 *	15.9 ± 7.6	33.0 ± 9.1 ‡	57.7 ± 14.3 ‡
LA-GCS (%)	20.2 ± 7.9	28.2 ± 8.7 *	25.7 ± 8.6 *	16.0 ± 5.5	26.7 ± 6.2 ‡	37.3 ± 9.5 ‡
LA-G3DS (%)	−0.4 ± 0.5	-7.1 ± 3.1 *	−17.2 ± 4.6 *,†	−4.6 ± 4.8	−7.9 ± 5.9 ‡	−8.6 ± 4.6 ‡
LA-GAS (%)	49.7 ± 23.5	72.4 ± 28.1 *	69.0 ± 26.3	29.9 ± 7.5	66.8 ± 15.1 ‡	116.5 ± 15.2 ‡
basal LV rotation (°)	−4.23 ± 1.78	4.16 ± 2.03	−4.77 ± 2.50	−4.36 ± 1.92	−4.28 ± 2.20	−4.07 ± 1.58
apical LV rotation (°)	10.50 ± 3.44	9.53 ± 3.54	8.12 ± 3.23 *	10.1 ± 3.9	9.35 ± 3.48	9.45 ± 3.28
LV twist (°)	14.73 ± 3.72	13.70 ± 3.65	12.88 ± 3.64	14.5 ± 3.7	13.63 ± 3.65	13.52 ± 3.78
time-to-LV twist (ms)	327 ± 105	342 ± 123	369 ± 176	358 ± 104	346 ± 144	319 ± 75

* $p < 0.05$ vs. LA-G3DS ≤ 1.75%; † $p < 0.05$ vs. 1.75% < LA-G3DS < 13.07%; ‡ $p < 0.05$ vs. LA-GAS ≤ 39.63%. Abbreviations. LA, left atrial; LV, left ventricular; G3DS, global three-dimensional strain; GAS, global area strain; GCS, global circumferential strain; GLS, global longitudinal strain; GRS, global radial strain.

3.6. Increased LA Peak Reservoir Strains and Basal and Apical LV Rotations

Only apical LV rotation proved to be significantly reduced in the case of the highest peak LA-G3DS. Other global LA peak reservoir strains did not show any associations with apical and basal rotations of the LV (Tables 3 and 4).

3.7. Feasibility of 3DSTE-Derived Measurements

The frame rate proved to be 31 ± 2 fps. This study comprised 308 healthy individuals, but 151 cases were excluded due to the image quality being insufficient for LA and/or LV quantifications. According to this fact, the overall feasibility proved to be 51%.

3.8. Reproducibility of 3DSTE-Derived Assessments

The mean ± SD difference in rotations of the LV base and apex and LA peak reservoir strains as assessed by 3DSTE simultaneously were assessed two times by the same observer and by two independent observers together with ICCs (Table 5).

Table 5. Intra- and inter-observer agreement for three-dimensional speckle-tracking echocardiography-derived apical and basal left ventricular rotations and left atrial peak reservoir strains in healthy adults.

	Intra-Observer Agreement		Inter-Observer Agreement	
	Mean ± 2SD Difference in Values Obtained by Two Measurements of the Same Observer	ICC Between Measurements of the Same Observer	Mean ± 2SD Difference in Values Obtained by 2 Measurements of the Same Observer	ICC Between Measurements of the Same Observer
Apical LV Rotation (°)	0.6 ± 0.4	0.81 ($p < 0.001$)	0.7 ± 0.7	0.80 ($p < 0.001$)
Basal LV Rotation (°)	0.3 ± 0.2	0.82 ($p < 0.001$)	0.3 ± 0.3	0.81 ($p < 0.001$)
LA-GRS (%)	−1.9 ± 11.1	0.86 ($p < 0.001$)	−4.0 ± 10.4	0.83 ($p < 0.001$)
LA-GLS (%)	4.7 ± 15.8	0.82 ($p < 0.001$)	4.9 ± 16.1	0.80 ($p < 0.001$)
LA-GCS (%)	3.1 ± 7.5	0.81 ($p < 0.001$)	3.6 ± 8.9	0.79 ($p < 0.001$)
LA-GAS (%)	6.7 ± 34.7	0.81 ($p < 0.001$)	11.1 ± 35.3	0.79 ($p < 0.001$)
LA-G3DS (%)	−1.3 ± 10.2	0.82 ($p < 0.001$)	−2.1 ± 9.4	0.80 ($p < 0.001$)

Abbreviations. LA = left atrial, LV = left ventricular, G3DS = global three-dimensional strain. GAS = global area strain, GCS = global circumferential strain, GLS = global longitudinal strain, GRS = global radial strain, ICC = interclass correlation coefficient.

4. Discussion

In left ventricular (LV) systole, the coordinated complex movement of heart chambers and valves is observed. Due to the spatial structure of the LV, its systolic pump function is the result of the coordinated work of the muscle fibers that make up the LV. However, due to the oblique muscle LV fibers running perpendicular to each other, not only can contraction be detected in systole, but the basal region of the LV rotates in the clockwise direction and the apical region of the LV rotates in the counterclockwise direction, having a specific 'towel-wringing' like movement, a phenomenon that is called LV twist. This sort of motion seems to be responsible for approximately 40% of ejection [3–7]. While the cavity of the LV is the smallest in end-systole, its walls thicken, narrow and shorten in the radial, circumferential and longitudinal directions, represented by specific LV strains. In the left atrium (LA), wall segments move in the opposite direction, ensuring reservoir function in systole. The LA cavity is the largest in end-systole, explaining why this phase is called 'reservoir', while thinning, lengthening and widening of the LA walls in the radial, longitudinal and circumferential directions represented by negative LA global radial strain (GRS) and positive LA global circumferential strain (GCS) and LA global longitudinal strain (GLS) are seen, respectively [1–3,8,9]. Due to the fact that the interaction of certain LV and LA features has not been deeply examined, to the best of the authors' knowledge, this is the first time where a three-dimensional (3D) speckle-tracking echocardiography (3DSTE)-derived analysis of the relationship between LV rotational mechanics and LA reservoir deformation represented by LA peak strains were performed in healthy adult volunteers to determine their relationship.

3DSTE seems to be an ideal method for the simultaneous analysis of LV rotational mechanics and LA deformation at the same time. 3DSTE is a non-invasive, non-radiating, easy-to-learn and easy-to-implement procedure, which can be performed several times within a relatively short time, even in healthy subjects. These advantages make it possible to perform physiological studies based on 3DSTE [10–13]. In the past, simultaneous routine 3D measurement of quantitative features of LV twist represented by apical and basal LV rotations and LA deformation represented by its strains could not be quantified, and only two-dimensional (2D)-projected parameters could be calculated in specific planes determined by the observer (1). This sort of approach of evaluation was based on certain predetermined assumptions, which could theoretically challenge the accuracy of the measurements (1). Therefore, according to recent recommendations, 2D speckle-tracking echocardiography (STE)-derived determination of LV rotational mechanics is not recommended, and only 3D echocardiography is suggested [10–14]. Although numerous studies have demonstrated the clinical possibility and importance of LA strain determination during 2DSTE, their 3DSTE-based determination seems to be closer to reality. In addition, 3DSTE is validated and normal reference values of LV rotational mechanics and LA strains measured in healthy subjects are also available [14–19].

In a recent study, strong associations between LA volumes and LV rotational mechanics were found [20]. The rotation of the LV base was highest in the presence of the highest maximum LA volume in end-systole (and the LA preatrial contraction volume in early diastole), and the rotation of the LV apex did not associate obviously with any LA volumes. End-systolic LA volume did not relate to LV rotations, but the highest end-systolic rotation of the LV base was associated with increased diastolic LA volumes, and reduced diastolic LA volumes were seen in the case of increased rotation of the LV apex. These findings could theoretically explain that blood flowing into the LV in diastole results in increased basal (not apical) LV rotation, as this region is closest to the LA outflow/LV inflow. End-systolic apical LV rotation was associated with lower volumes of the LA, suggesting that it may play a role in lower atrial preload [20].

With the presented findings, our knowledge was extended with several facts. The highest rotation of the LV base was associated with the lowest LA-GCS (LA widening) and LA-GAS. Moreover, with higher apical LV rotation, lower LA-GRS (LA thinning) and LA-G3DS were associated. With increasing LA peak reservoir strains, neither basal nor apical LV rotations showed associations except for the rotation of the LV apex, which was lowest in the presence of the highest LA-G3DS.

To determine the clinical importance of a phenomenon in a specific abnormality, better understanding in healthy circumstances has a significant importance. The presented results suggest a complex adaptation to changes in the volumes and functional properties of the LA and LV, suggesting that each left heart chamber can affect the other, even in healthy circumstances. It must also be noted that certain parameters (volumes, functional characteristics, etc.) are not independent of each other, so they must be examined together, which can make analysis very complicated. Therefore, further multi-parameter investigations are warranted in healthy subjects. Moreover, similar studies are also needed to examine these relationships in certain pathologies, which are associated with changes in LA and/or LV morphology and function. Future studies examining patients with early systolic LV abnormalities (e.g., cases with reduced LV-GLS but preserved LV ejection fraction) would be worthwhile to investigate which relationship/association disappears the earliest and which still exists in healthy subjects based on the present research. This sort of analysis could help us form a deeper understanding of the development of the early stages of heart failure.

During this study's analyses, many factors were not taken account in order to highlight the most important ones, e.g., the roles of age, gender difference, heart rate and blood pressure were not investigated. Accordingly, an even more complex approach would be necessary to understand the presented physiological associations.

5. Limitations

The limitations presented as follows were the most important ones of this study.

Firstly, the sample size could have been larger to allow analyses like the evaluation of gender differences or subjects being in different age decades.

According to a consensus document, measurement of global LA strain is recommended and radial (or transverse) strain is not recommended. However, due to the experimental nature of this analysis, a full analysis was performed [21].

Image quality was an important aspect. Under current technical conditions, 2D echocardiography still has a significant advantage, which limits the usability of 3DSTE. In the present study, the overall feasibility proved to be only 51%. Further improvements are needed to improve the temporal and spatial resolution of the images taken [10–13,22].

3DSTE is capable of evaluating LV strain parameters simultaneously using the same 3D echocardiography dataset. A detailed analysis of LV/LA strains would have exceeded the limits of the present paper and could well be the subject of another study.

This study did not purpose to assess associations between LA volumes and LV rotational mechanics due to the detailed investigation of this topic [20].

The validation of calculated parameters was not among the objectives of the current study due to their validated nature [15–18].

The pulmonary veins and the LA appendage were excluded from the evaluations.

Morphological abnormalities of the LA were not aimed to be characterized.

3DSTE-derived evaluation of the volumes and functional properties of other heart chambers were not to be performed either.

In this study, analyses were performed with the atrial septum as part of the LA.

Finally, both parameters of LV rotational mechanics and LA strains had specific age and gender dependencies, which could have affected the findings [14,19].

6. Conclusions

In LV systole, LV rotational mechanics is associated with LA deformation, represented by LA peak reservoir strains even in healthy circumstances. While basal LV rotation is associated with LA widening, apical LV rotation is associated with LA thinning, suggesting the close cooperation of the LV and LA in systole even in healthy adults.

Author Contributions: A.N.: Conceptualization, writing—original draft and writing—review and editing. Á.K.: Methodology, investigation and data curation. N.A.: Writing—review and editing. C.L.: Resources. All authors have read and agreed to the published version of the manuscript.

Funding: This research received no external funding.

Institutional Review Board Statement: The authors take responsibility for all aspects of the reliability and freedom from bias of the data presented and their discussed interpretation (Registration No.: 71/2011).

Informed Consent Statement: Informed consent was obtained from all individual participants included in this study.

Data Availability Statement: The manuscript has not been published elsewhere. Data are contained within the article.

Conflicts of Interest: The authors declare no conflicts of interest.

References

1. Lang, R.M.; Badano, L.P.; Mor-Avi, V.; Afilalo, J.; Armstrong, A.; Ernande, L.; Flachskampf, F.A.; Foster, E.; Goldstein, S.A.; Kuznetsova, T.; et al. Recommendations for cardiac chamber quantification by echocardiography in adults: An update from the American Society of Echocardiography and the European Association of Cardiovascular Imaging. *Eur. Heart J. Cardiovasc. Imaging* **2015**, *16*, 233–270. [CrossRef] [PubMed]
2. Narang, A.; Addetia, K. An introduction to left ventricular strain. *Curr. Opin. Cardiol.* **2018**, *33*, 455–463. [CrossRef] [PubMed]
3. Nakatani, S. Left ventricular rotation and twist: Why should we learn? *J. Cardiovasc. Ultrasound* **2011**, *19*, 1–6. [CrossRef] [PubMed]
4. Bloechlinger, S.; Grander, W.; Bryner, J.; Dünser, M.W. Left ventricular rotation: A neglected aspect of the cardiac cycle. *Intensive Care Med.* **2011**, *37*, 156–163. [CrossRef] [PubMed]
5. Omar, A.M.S.; Vallabhajosyula, S.; Sengupta, P.P. Left Ventricular Twist and Torsion. Research Observations and Clinical Applications. *Circ. Cardiovasc. Imaging* **2015**, *8*, e003029. [CrossRef]

6. Sengupta, P.P.; Tajik, A.J.; Chandrasekaran, K.; Khandheria, B.K. Twist mechanics of the left ventricle: Principles and application. *JACC Cardiovasc. Imaging* **2008**, *1*, 366–376. [CrossRef]
7. Stöhr, E.J.; Shave, R.E.; Baggish, A.L.; Weiner, R.B. Left ventricular twist mechanics in the context of normal physiology and cardiovascular disease: A review of studies using speckle tracking echocardiography. *Am. J. Physiol. Heart Circ. Physiol.* **2016**, *311*, H633–H644. [CrossRef]
8. Blume, G.G.; Mcleod, C.J.; Barnes, M.E.; Seward, J.B.; Pellikka, P.A.; Bastiansen, P.M.; Tsang, T.S.M. Left atrial function: Physiology, assessment, and clinical implications. *Eur. J. Echocardiogr.* **2011**, *12*, 421–430. [CrossRef]
9. Seward, J.B.; Hebl, V.B. Left atrial anatomy and physiology: Echo/Doppler assessment. *Curr. Opin. Cardiol.* **2014**, *29*, 403–407. [CrossRef]
10. Ammar, K.A.; Paterick, T.E.; Khandheria, B.K.; Jan, M.F.; Kramer, C.; Umland, M.M.; Tercius, A.J.; Baratta, L.; Tajik, A.J. Myocardial mechanics: Understanding and applying three-dimensional speckle tracking echocardiography in clinical practice. *Echocardiography* **2012**, *29*, 861–872. [CrossRef]
11. Urbano-Moral, J.A.; Patel, A.R.; Maron, M.S.; Arias-Godinez, J.A.; Pandian, N.G. Three-dimensional speckle-tracking echocardiography: Methodological aspects and clinical potential. *Echocardiography* **2012**, *29*, 997–1010. [CrossRef] [PubMed]
12. Muraru, D.; Niero, A.; Rodriguez-Zanella, H.; Cherata, D.; Badano, L. Three-dimensional speckle-tracking echocardiography: Benefits and limitations of integrating myocardial mechanics with three-dimensional imaging. *Cardiovasc. Diagn. Ther.* **2018**, *8*, 101–117. [CrossRef] [PubMed]
13. Gao, L.; Lin, Y.; Ji, M.; Wu, W.; Li, H.; Qian, M.; Zhang, L.; Xie, M.; Li, Y. Clinical Utility of Three-Dimensional Speckle-Tracking Echocardiography in Heart Failure. *J. Clin. Med.* **2022**, *11*, 6307. [CrossRef] [PubMed]
14. Kormányos, Á.; Kalapos, A.; Domsik, P.; Lengyel, C.; Forster, T.; Nemes, A. Normal values of left ventricular rotational parameters in healthy adults—Insights from the three-dimensional speckle tracking echocardiographic MAGYAR-Healthy Study. *Echocardiography* **2019**, *36*, 714–721. [CrossRef]
15. Ashraf, M.; Myronenko, A.; Nguyen, T.; Inage, A.; Smith, W.; Lowe, R.I.; Thiele, K.; Gibbons Kroeker, C.A.; Tyberg, J.V.; Smallhorn, J.F.; et al. Defining left ventricular apex-to-base twist mechanics computed from high-resolution 3D echocardiography: Validation against sonomicrometry. *JACC Cardiovasc. Imaging* **2010**, *3*, 227–234. [CrossRef]
16. Zhou, Z.; Ashraf, M.; Hu, D.; Dai, X.; Xu, Y.; Kenny, B.; Cameron, B.; Nguyen, T.; Xiong, L.; Sahn, D.J. Three-dimensional speckle-tracking imaging for left ventricular rotation measurement: An in vitro validation study. *J. Ultrasound. Med.* **2010**, *29*, 903–909. [CrossRef]
17. Andrade, J.; Cortez, L.D.; Campos, O.; Arruda, A.L.; Pinheiro, J.; Vulcanis, L.; Shiratsuchi, T.S.; Kalil-Filho, R.; Cerri, G.G. Left ventricular twist: Comparison between two- and three-dimensional speckle-tracking echocardiography in healthy volunteers. *Eur. J. Echocardiogr.* **2011**, *12*, 76–79. [CrossRef]
18. Nagaya, M.; Kawasaki, M.; Tanaka, R.; Onishi, N.; Sato, N.; Ono, K.; Watanabe, T.; Minatoguchi, S.; Miwa, H.; Goto, Y.; et al. Quantitative validation of left atrial structure and function by two-dimensional and three-dimensional speckle tracking echocardiography: A comparative study with three-dimensional computed tomography. *J. Cardiol.* **2013**, *62*, 188–194. [CrossRef]
19. Nemes, A.; Kormányos, Á.; Domsik, P.; Kalapos, A.; Lengyel, C.; Forster, T. Normal reference values of three-dimensional speckle-tracking echocardiography-derived left atrial strain parameters (results from the MAGYAR-Healthy Study). *Int. J. Cardiovasc. Imaging* **2019**, *35*, 991–998. [CrossRef]
20. Nemes, A.; Kormányos, Á.; Ruzsa, Z.; Achim, A.; Ambrus, N.; Lengyel, C. Dependence of Left Ventricular Rotational Mechanics on Left Atrial Volumes in Non-Smoker Healthy Adults: Analysis Based on the Three-Dimensional Speckle-Tracking Echocardiographic MAGYAR-Healthy Study. *J. Clin. Med.* **2023**, *12*, 1235. [CrossRef]
21. Badano, L.P.; Kolias, T.J.; Muraru, D.; Abraham, T.P.; Aurigemma, G.; Edvardsen, T.; D'Hooge, J.; Donal, E.; Fraser, A.G.; Marwick, T.; et al. Standardization of left atrial, right ventricular, and right atrial deformation imaging using two-dimensional speckle tracking echocardiography: A consensus document of the EACVI/ASE/Industry Task Force to standardize deformation imaging. *Eur. Heart J. Cardiovasc. Imaging* **2018**, *19*, 591–600. [CrossRef] [PubMed]
22. Lang, R.M.; Addetia, K.; Narang, A.; Mor-Avi, V. 3-dimensional echocardiography: Latest developments and future directions. *JACC Cardiovasc Imaging.* **2018**, *11*, 1854–1878. [CrossRef] [PubMed]

biomedicines

MDPI

Review

Cancer Therapy-Related Cardiac Dysfunction: A Review of Current Trends in Epidemiology, Diagnosis, and Treatment

Panagiotis Theofilis [1], Panayotis K. Vlachakis [1], Evangelos Oikonomou [2], Maria Drakopoulou [1], Paschalis Karakasis [3], Anastasios Apostolos [1], Konstantinos Pamporis [1], Konstantinos Tsioufis [1] and Dimitris Tousoulis [1,*]

[1] 1st Department of Cardiology, Hippokration General Hospital, National and Kapodistrian University of Athens, 11527 Athens, Greece; panos.theofilis@hotmail.com (P.T.); vlachakispanag@gmail.com (P.K.V.); mdrakopoulou@med.uoa.gr (M.D.); anastasisapostolos@gmail.com (A.A.); konstantinospab@gmail.com (K.P.); ktsioufis@gmail.com (K.T.)

[2] 3rd Department of Cardiology, Thoracic Diseases General Hospital Sotiria, National and Kapodistrian University of Athens, 11527 Athens, Greece; boikono@gmail.com

[3] 2nd Department of Cardiology, Hippokration General Hospital, Aristotle University of Thessaloniki, 54642 Thessaloniki, Greece; pakar15@hotmail.com

[*] Correspondence: drtousoulis@hotmail.com

Abstract: Cancer therapy-related cardiac dysfunction (CTRCD) has emerged as a significant concern with the rise of effective cancer treatments like anthracyclines and targeted therapies such as trastuzumab. While these therapies have improved cancer survival rates, their unintended cardiovascular side effects can lead to heart failure, cardiomyopathy, and arrhythmias. The pathophysiology of CTRCD involves oxidative stress, mitochondrial dysfunction, and calcium dysregulation, resulting in irreversible damage to cardiomyocytes. Inflammatory cytokines, disrupted growth factor signaling, and coronary atherosclerosis further contribute to this dysfunction. Advances in cardio-oncology have led to the early detection of CTRCD using cardiac biomarkers like troponins and imaging techniques such as echocardiography and cardiac magnetic resonance (CMR). These tools help identify asymptomatic patients at risk of cardiac events before the onset of clinical symptoms. Preventive strategies, including the use of cardioprotective agents like beta-blockers, angiotensin-converting enzyme inhibitors, mineralocorticoid receptor antagonists, and sodium-glucose cotransporter-2 inhibitors have shown promise in reducing the incidence of CTRCD. This review summarizes the mechanisms, detection methods, and emerging treatments for CTRCD, emphasizing the importance of interdisciplinary collaboration between oncologists and cardiologists to optimize care and improve both cancer and cardiovascular outcomes.

Keywords: cancer; cancer treatment-related cardiac dysfunction; global longitudinal strain; cardiac magnetic resonance; cardio-oncology

1. Introduction

The improvement in oncology care, particularly through the use of potent pharmacotherapies like anthracyclines and targeted agents such as trastuzumab, has dramatically enhanced cancer survival rates. However, these advances come with a significant risk: cancer therapy-related cardiac toxicity (CTRCD). As cancer treatments become more effective, their unintended cardiovascular side effects have become a critical issue. Indeed, while significant advances have been achieved in reducing cancer-related mortality, an increase in cardiovascular mortality is noted beyond the first years of cancer diagnosis [1].

Chemotherapeutic agents like anthracyclines generate reactive oxygen species (ROS), leading to oxidative stress and irreversible damage to cardiomyocytes [2]. Similarly, anti-vascular endothelial growth factor (VEGF) therapies used in treating solid tumors can cause hypertension and myocardial hypoperfusion, increasing the risk of heart failure (HF). With the emergence of powerful drugs, patients are often faced with the dual challenge of managing cancer while protecting cardiovascular health. Cardio-oncology, an interdisciplinary field that bridges oncology and cardiology, has become essential in managing this delicate balance. Early detection of cardiotoxicity through biomarkers like troponins and imaging modalities such as echocardiography and cardiac magnetic resonance (CMR) plays a pivotal role in identifying cardiovascular risks before irreversible damage occurs.

In response to the increasing prevalence of CTRCD, there is a growing focus on preventive and therapeutic strategies, including the use of cardioprotective agents like beta-blockers, angiotensin-converting enzyme (ACE) inhibitors, and angiotensin receptor blockers. These medications, when initiated early, can help mitigate the cardiovascular side effects of cancer therapy, allowing patients to continue potentially life-saving treatments. As the field of cardio-oncology continues to evolve, the goal is to optimize cancer treatment while minimizing its cardiovascular impact, ensuring both improved survival and quality of life for cancer patients. In this review, we summarize the existing evidence in the pathophysiology, epidemiology, and management of CTRCD. While multiple cancer therapies are associated with cardiac dysfunction, this review concerns mostly therapies with the most robust evidence for CTRCD, including anthracyclines, HER2-targeted therapies like trastuzumab, and anti-VEGF agents. These therapies are prioritized due to their widespread use and significant cardiovascular impact in clinical practice.

2. Definition

Cardiovascular toxicities related to cancer therapies encompass a broad spectrum of conditions that affect the heart and vascular system. These manifestations necessitate cross-disciplinary communication to effectively describe cardiovascular events and integrate these standards into routine clinical practice and research. The recently published 2022 ESC Guidelines for the management of cardio-oncology, endorsed by the Scientific Council of the International Cardio-Oncology Society (IC-OS), provide comprehensive definitions of these toxicities [3].

More specifically, "Cancer Therapy-Related Cardiac Dysfunction" (CTRCD) is defined as the adverse impact on cardiac structure and function in cancer patients, presenting as either asymptomatic cardiac dysfunction or symptomatic HF related to the therapy received. Confirmation of CTRCD includes any of the following: a reduction in left ventricular ejection fraction (LVEF), symptoms of congestive heart failure, signs associated with heart failure (such as S3 gallop or tachycardia), or a reduction in LVEF from baseline by 5–10%. Symptomatic CTRCD is characterized by a HF syndrome with typical symptoms and signs of volume overload or inadequate perfusion caused by structural and functional abnormalities of the heart consistent with AHA/ACC Stage C/D HF. In contrast, asymptomatic CTRCD is more common during cancer therapy and is often identified through changes in LVEF on screening echocardiograms during treatment or as an incidental finding during survivorship surveillance [4].

The guidelines also define various manifestations of cancer therapy-related cardiac toxicity. Cardiomyopathy and HF are significant conditions that can arise, with myocarditis often resulting from direct toxicity or immune-mediated events in cancer patients. Vascular toxicity, characterized by arterial occlusion due to blood clots, can lead to luminal obstruction and reduced blood flow through altered vascular reactivity, thrombosis, atherosclerosis, or vasculitis, and can be either clinically silent or symptomatic. Hypertension in cancer patients may be temporary and treatment-induced, with a more abrupt onset that can lead to end-organ damage and other complications. Uncontrolled hypertension may necessitate the cessation of cancer treatment, significantly impacting the patient's oncologic care. Finally, several cancer therapies have been recognized to cause QTc prolongation, including arsenic trioxide, HDAC inhibitors, tyrosine kinase inhibitors (e.g., vandetanib, vemurafenib, ceritinib, gilteritinib, trametinib, and those targeting BCR-Abl and the VEGF signaling pathway), and Cyclin-dependent kinase (CDK) 4–6 inhibitors [4].

Understanding these definitions and mechanisms is crucial, as "speaking the same language" among clinicians could improve the management of cardiovascular health in cancer patients and ensure optimal therapeutic outcomes.

3. Epidemiology

The epidemiology of cardiotoxicity varies significantly depending on the population studied and the specific agents involved. In oncology, the incidence of cardiotoxicity is influenced by the type of chemotherapeutic agent, cumulative dose, combination therapies, and individual patient risk factors such as age, pre-existing cardiovascular disease, and genetic predispositions.

Specifically, the prevalence of late symptomatic anthracycline-induced cardiotoxicity varies widely, influenced by patient age, anthracycline dose, cancer type, cardiovascular risk factors, pre-existing heart disease, and follow-up duration [5]. In adults, symptomatic HF typically appears within two to three years after anthracycline treatment [6]. A study of 135 patients with non-Hodgkin lymphoma showed that 20% experienced significant cardiac events within a year of anthracycline therapy [7]. Asymptomatic LV dysfunction is more common than symptomatic disease, with rates ranging from 7% (LVEF) to 45% (cardiac strain) [8]. A trial on statin therapy in doxorubicin-treated patients showed a decrease in LVEF from 63% to 57% over 24 months [9]. In an echocardiographic study of 1853 adult childhood cancer survivors, 7% had asymptomatic LVEF reduction below 50% [10]. A CMR imaging study reported a 14% prevalence of reduced LVEF in 114 adult childhood cancer survivors [11]. Another CMR study found 26% of adults treated with low to moderate anthracycline doses had an asymptomatic LVEF reduction below 50% at six months [12]. A Kaiser study linked anthracycline therapy for breast cancer to a 1.84-fold increased risk of cardiomyopathy/HF and a 2.91-fold increased risk of cardiovascular mortality [13]. In children, cardiotoxicity is often detected long after exposure, particularly in childhood cancer survivors, who have a nearly 6-fold higher risk of HF compared to siblings, mainly due to anthracycline exposure [10].

The incidence of trastuzumab-related cardiotoxicity varies based on patient factors such as previous chemotherapy, pre-existing heart disease, and age. While the risk of HF or cardiomyopathy with trastuzumab is low, it can be mitigated by limiting cumulative anthracycline doses to below 300 mg/m^2. Nevertheless, close cardiac monitoring is necessary [14]. In large randomized trials of adjuvant trastuzumab for HER2-positive breast cancer, which included stringent cardiac monitoring and limited anthracycline doses, a modest incidence of cardiotoxicity was observed [15–17]. A 2012 meta-analysis of these trials, involving 11,991 women, found that trastuzumab-treated patients had an increased risk of severe HF (2.5% vs. 0.4%; RR 5.11) and a reduction in LVEF (RR 1.83). The cardiotoxicity profile was similar regardless of whether chemotherapy and trastuzumab were administered concurrently or sequentially. Shorter treatment periods did not significantly increase HF risk [18]. A subsequent study of around 400 patients treated with paclitaxel and trastuzumab for node-negative disease reported even lower cardiotoxicity rates, with only 0.5% developing grade 3 left ventricular systolic dysfunction and 3% experiencing asymptomatic LVEF decline. These findings compare favorably with older trials involving higher doses of concurrent doxorubicin [19,20].

The incidence of fluorouracil (FU)-related cardiotoxicity ranges from 1% to 19%, with most reports indicating a risk of 8% or less [21]. This variability is likely due to differences in defining cardiotoxicity, FU administration methods, underlying coronary artery disease (CAD), concurrent radiation therapy or anthracyclines, and monitoring intensity. The highest rates are seen in closely monitored patients. For instance, a study of 102 patients receiving FU, monitored with ECG, echocardiography, and radionuclide ventriculography, found 19% experienced reversible angina pectoris within 24 h of starting FU, often with accompanying ECG changes [22]. Asymptomatic ECG changes, arrhythmias, and elevated NT-proBNP levels during FU chemotherapy suggest possible subclinical cardiotoxicity, though the clinical significance is uncertain [22–24].

Tyrosine kinase inhibitors (TKIs) are associated with significant cardiovascular toxicity, affecting both the heart and vascular system [25]. Adverse effects are observed in single- and multi-targeted TKIs, particularly through mechanisms such as VEGF inhibition, which impairs angiogenesis and myocardial perfusion and leads to microvascular dysfunction [25]. Myocardial dysfunction and HF are common, with a meta-analysis of clinical studies in 10,670 patients reporting an incidence of asymptomatic LV dysfunction at 2.4%, while VEGF inhibitors like sunitinb and sorafenib are linked to progressive HF [26]. Specifically, VEGF inhibitors can reduce capillary rarefaction (myocardial capillary network) and impaired myocardial contractility [27]. Anti-HER2 TKIs, such as lapatinib, show higher cardiotoxicity rates in metastatic settings, with HF reported in 3% of patients with breast cancer [28]. HTN is another prevalent side effect, which is seen in 30–80% of patients on VEGFIs and in up to 78.3% of those treated with ibrutinib [25,29]. QTc prolongation occurs in 0.1% of VEGF-inhibitor cases but is higher with third-generation EGFR TKIs such as osimertinib [30,31]. Finaly, thromboembolic events are associated with VEGF inhibitors, with arterial thrombosis reported in 1.7% and 1.4% of patients on sorafenib and sunitinib, respectively [25,32].

Immune checkpoint inhibitors (ICIs) are associated with rare but significant cardiotoxicity, primarily presenting as myocarditis. A retrospective study across eight clinical centers found a myocarditis prevalence of 1.14% [33]. In a phase II trial with pembrolizumab for thymic epithelial tumors, 34% of patients experienced grade 3 or higher immune-related adverse events, including 9% with myocarditis and 6% with myasthenia gravis [34]. Combination ICI therapy increases myocarditis risk to 1.33%, compared to 0.31% for monotherapy [35]. Myocarditis typically manifests within the first three months, with most cases occurring within six weeks of treatment, and combination therapy-related myocarditis shows a higher mortality rate (67%) compared to monotherapy (36%) [36]. Other CV complications include a 1% incidence of myocardial infarction in lung cancer patients treated with ICIs and tachyarrhythmias, bradyarrhythmias, and prolonged QTc, indicating an elevated risk of ventricular arrhythmias [37,38].

4. Pathophysiology

The pathophysiology of cardiotoxicity involves complex mechanisms that result in myocardial damage (Table 1, Figure 1). For chemotherapeutic agents like anthracyclines, the primary mechanism is believed to be the generation of ROS leading to oxidative stress, mitochondrial dysfunction, and subsequent cardiomyocyte apoptosis [39]. In cardiomyocytes, which have abundant mitochondria, ROS levels increase during chemotherapy, predominantly producing superoxide anions [40]. Due to their short half-life, ROS primarily affect the mitochondria that generate them [41]. Additionally, the heart's crucial antioxidant systems, which neutralize free radicals, are diminished [42]. This includes reduced complex I activity and decreased levels of cardiolipin, a phospholipid essential for the function of anion carriers and electron transport complexes, as well as for enhancing cytochrome oxidase activity [43]. Cardiolipin, an unsaturated fatty acid vital for electron transport and cytochrome oxidase activity, is prone to peroxidation, leading to decreased cytochrome c oxidase activity and increased oxidative stress [44]. Oxidative stress in the cardiac muscle can lead to altered gene expression, calcium overload, cellular hypertrophy, ventricular remodeling, and cell death via apoptosis. These pathological changes can result in cardiomyopathy and HF [40].

Table 1. Mechanisms of cancer therapy-related cardiac dysfunction (CTRCD).

Mechanism	Drug Class	Observed Symptoms	Key Processes	References
Oxidative Stress	Anthracyclines	Cardiomyopathy, heart failure	ROS generation, mitochondrial dysfunction, cardiomyocyte apoptosis	[39,40,43,44]
Inflammation	Immune checkpoint inhibitors	Myocarditis, arrhythmias	Cytokine storm, IL-1β and IL-6 mediated ion channel alterations, QT prolongation	[45–47]
Calcium Overload	Anthracyclines, TKIs	Ventricular arrhythmias, myocardial injury	Disruption of calcium regulation, increased diastolic calcium levels, RYR2 dysfunction	[48–50]
VEGF	Anti-VEGF therapies	Hypertension, myocardial ischemia	Endothelial dysfunction, impaired angiogenesis, microvascular dysfunction	[27,51,52]
Pyroptosis	Immune checkpoint inhibitors	Myocardial necrosis, inflammation	Caspase and gasdermin activation, increased cytokine release during ischemia–reperfusion injury	[53]
Fibrosis	HER2-targeted therapies	Myocardial stiffening, heart failure	Increased fibroblast activation, extracellular matrix remodeling, TGF-β pathway activation	[12,54]

ROS: reactive oxygen species, IL: interleukin, TKI: tyrosine kinase inhibitor, VEGF: vascular endothelial growth factor, RYR2: ryanodine receptor 2.

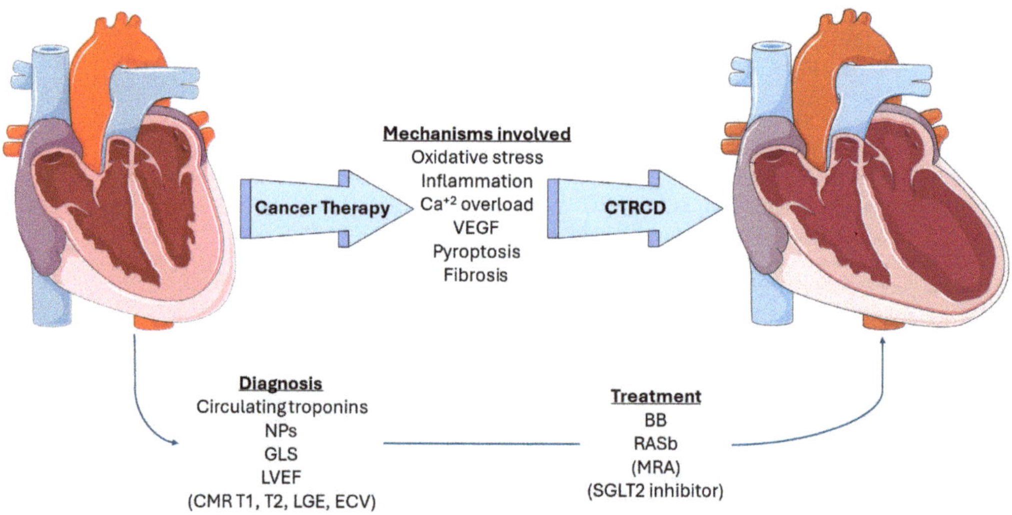

Figure 1. Overview of pathophysiologic mechanisms, diagnosis, and treatment of CTRCD. Content in parenthesis represents potential approaches that have not been incorporated into guidelines. VEGF: vascular endothelial growth factor, NP: natriuretic peptide, GLS: global longitudinal strain, LVEF: left ventricular ejection fraction, CMR: cardiac magnetic resonance, LGE: late gadolinium enhancement, ECV: extracellular volume, BB: beta blocker, RASb: renin-angiotensin system blocker, MRA: mineralocorticoid receptor antagonist, and SGLT2: sodium-glucose cotransporter-2.

Moreover, chronic inflammation and cytokine storming, often perpetuated by malignancy and chemotherapy, could have deleterious effects on the cardiovascular system. Inflammatory cytokines such as Interleukin (IL)-1β and IL-6 alter cardiac ion channel function, increasing the risk of arrhythmias and sudden cardiac death [45]. For instance, increased inflammatory markers inhibit human ether-a-go-go (hERG)-related channel, reducing the rapid delayed rectifier current (IKr), prolonging the QT interval and action potential duration, and heightening the risk of ventricular arrhythmias like Torsades de Pointes [46,47]. Key ion channels, including SERCA2 and Cav1.2 (L-type Ca^{2+} channels), are affected by elevated levels of IL-6 and IL-1 [55]. Chronic exposure to IL-6 has been shown to decrease SERCA2 activity, impairing Ca^{2+} reuptake and leading to prolonged Ca^{2+} exposure, sustained excitation, and an increased risk of arrhythmias [56,57]. Additionally, IL-6 plays a complex role in myocardial contractility [58]. While acute IL-6 exposure can help preserve myocardial function, chronic exposure can lead to pathological changes, including immune cell infiltration and increased connective tissue production. Continuous IL-6 and IL-6 receptor expression can cause persistent gp130 signaling, promoting left ventricular hypertrophy and cardiomyopathy [59]. STAT-3, a downstream target of IL-6, is implicated in cardiac hypertrophy, while tumor necrosis factor (TNF)-α has been observed to reduce ejection fraction and induce HF in animal studies [58,60]. IL-1β and IL-18 also promote apoptosis by increasing caspase and gasdermin activity, contributing to myocardial pyroptosis, a form of necrosis associated with excessive cytokine release during ischemia–reperfusion injury [53].

Calcium regulation within the myocardium is crucial for muscle contractility and conduction in the atrioventricular and sinoatrial nodes. Excess calcium can lead to increased firing of these nodes, and any pathological alterations in calcium handling can result in cardiotoxicity, which is a known mechanism of chemotherapy-induced cardiotoxicity. Certain chemotherapeutic drugs significantly affect calcium homeostasis in cardiac tissue. Studies suggest that these drugs increase ROS levels, which subsequently cause calcium overload [48]. For instance, doxorubicin has been shown to increase diastolic calcium overload in rat cardiac myocytes by promoting calcium leakage from the sarcoplasmic reticulum through modulation of Ca/calmodulin-dependent protein kinase II (CaMKII) activity [49]. Lowering ROS levels, reducing Na^{+}/Ca^{2+} exchanger expression, and preventing CaMKII hyperphosphorylation can mitigate anthracycline-induced myocardial fibrosis [61]. Excess calcium can lead to fatal atrial and ventricular arrhythmias, with common ECG findings of early and delayed afterdepolarizations. Calcium overload, often due to ryanodine receptor 2 (RYR2) dysfunction, can create ectopic foci and reentry circuits, disrupting cardiac conduction [50].

Growth factors are essential for cell proliferation and integrity. VEGF supports angiogenesis, myocardial regeneration, and stress response by upregulating nitric oxide, which inhibits platelet adhesion and acts as a vasodilator [51]. However, VEGF also promotes tumor growth and metastasis, leading to the use of anti-VEGF therapies in cancers like breast, lung, and colorectal cancer. Anti-VEGF drugs can cause significant cardiotoxicity, with up to 70% of patients developing arterial hypertension [52]. This is possibly due to increased endothelin-1 levels and higher systolic blood pressure, which can lead to cardiac remodeling, LV hypertrophy, diastolic dysfunction, and HF. Similarly, inhibiting platelet-derived growth factors (PDGFR) with drugs like sunitinib can cause hypertrophy and fibrosis [54]. Epidermal growth factor receptor inhibitors (EGFRis) also contribute to cardiotoxicity, with some patients experiencing severe HF when treated with herceptin and anthracyclines. Despite their benefits, the cardiotoxicity of anti-growth signaling therapies limits their use [62].

Finally, several chemotherapeutic drugs are implicated in atherosclerosis of the coronary arteries. Antimetabolites, antimicrotubule agents, and tyrosine kinase inhibitors commonly cause coronary artery disease due to alterations in signaling pathways and subsequent vasoconstrictive effects. VEGF inhibitors can lead to coronary artery occlusion and angina by reducing NO synthase activity via the Akt/PKB pathway, resulting in abnormal vascular tone and coagulation, especially during oxidative stress [27]. Combined with the increased coagulative tendency and the effects of radiotherapy in malignancy, these factors may significantly impact cardiovascular health and quality of life in cancer patients.

5. The Role of Biomarkers and Imaging in CTRCD

Biomarkers of cardiac dysfunction are crucial in the detection and subsequent management of CTRCD (Table 2). Early studies have shown that a rise in TnT following anticancer therapy (chemotherapy or radiotherapy) was associated with the incidence of CTRCD and is usually dose dependent [63,64]. According to a meta-analysis of eight studies (1294 patients receiving anticancer therapy), an increase in TnT at 3–6 months after the initiation of treatment was an strong predictor of CTRCD (area under receiver operating characteristics curve 0.90) [65]. It is therefore unsurprising that a rise in troponin irrespective of symptoms could indicate the presence of mild, asymptomatic CTRCD, according to the guidelines, and should be ordered in all patients prior to the initiation of anticancer therapy, even in those in the lowest risk categories.

Table 2. Circulating and novel imaging biomarkers in CTRCD.

Biomarker	Anticancer Therapy	Study Population	Outcomes	Ref
Hs-cTnT	Platinum and taxane-doublet chemotherapy with radiation of at least 60 Gy	190 patients with NSCLC	• Hs-cTnT increased from 4th week • Greater increase in left-sided tumors • Δhs-cTnT correlated with mean heart dose • Risk of cardiac adverse events higher if baseline hs-cTnT >10 ng/L (HR 4.06) or Δ-hs-cTnT >5 ng/L (HR 3.57)	[63]
Hs-cTnT	Not specified	930 patients attending the cardio-oncology outpatient clinic	• hs-cTnT above the median (≥7 ng/L) was an independent marker of all-cause mortality (OR 2.21)	[64]
CT-derived EAT volume index	Adjuvant AC ± Trastuzumab	41 breast cancer patients	• The EAT volume index was significantly higher in both groups at follow-up compared to baseline	[66]
CT-derived ECV	Neoadjuvant chemotherapy	102 breast cancer patients	• Development of CTRCD was associated with an increase in mean ECV after approximately 12 months, which had subsided at 5 years	[67]
Myocardial T2	Anthracycline	29 breast cancer patients	• Gradual increase of T2 values during chemotherapy	[68]
T1, T2, and ECV	Anthracycline + Trastuzumab	136 breast cancer patients	• Changes in ventricular volumes were associated with a change in T1, T2, and/or ECV • No significant associations were seen between any of the CMR tissue biomarkers and LVEF, GLS, or LVMi • Larger increase in T1, T2, and ECV was associated with a larger increase in BNP	[69]
CMR-LGE	Ibrutinib	49 cancer patients	• Native T1 and presence of LGE were higher in treated patients and were associated with the development of MACE (LGE HR: 4.9, T1 HR: 3.3)	[70]

Regarding imaging modalities, it is clear that echocardiography remains a first-line imaging modality in assessing CTRCD, either through the use of GLS or LVEF, as proposed by the existing guidelines, since it is a cost-effective and reproducible method. Recently, CMR has flourished in this field due to its ability in myocardial tissue characterization and detection of myocardial inflammation and fibrosis.

Changes in epicardial adipose tissue could be an early indicator of incident adverse cardiac remodeling, as shown in a previous study [71]. Chest computed tomography (CT) in patients receiving cardiotoxic chemotherapy has shown an expansion in the volume of epicardial adipose tissue [66]. Therefore, future studies will determine whether this imaging modality can detect patients at risk of CTRCD at an earlier stage and prompt cardioprotective treatment initiation. CT-derived myocardial extracellular volume could also present an appealing marker which requires further validation, since a small-scale study in 82 breast cancer patients found it to be an informative marker [67].

Cardiac magnetic resonance (CMR) has recently gained ground regarding the early recognition of CTRCD. A study evaluated the early detection of anthracycline-induced cardiotoxicity in breast cancer survivors using T2 CMR [68]. It revealed that myocardial T2, which indicates inflammation, increases after anthracycline therapy, preceding fibrosis and a decline in LVEF. Though LVEF remained stable initially, 35% of patients showed a significant drop in LVEF at follow-up, suggesting T2 as an early marker of cardiotoxicity. In another study in women undergoing breast cancer therapy with anthracyclines and trastuzumab, CMR markers of myocardial hyperemia and edema (relative myocardial enhancement, native T1, extracellular volume) increased after anthracycline chemotherapy or 3 months after trastuzumab treatment, indicating an inflammatory process during this period [69]. Moreover, they were associated with increased LV volumes and BNP levels but the changes were transient and not associated with the incidence of CTRCD. For cancer patients treated with ibrutinib for a median of 14 months, CMR late gadolinium enhancement (LGE) was present in 13.3% and indices of subclinical myocardial inflammation and fibrosis were found to be elevated in 63% and 28.6% of patients, respectively [70]. Interestingly, LGE (HR: 4.9; $p = 0.04$) and native-T1 (HR: 3.3; $p = 0.05$) were predictive of incident adverse cardiovascular events (atrial fibrillation, heart failure, symptomatic ventricular arrhythmias, and sudden death). We should note that according to a study in 125 women with HER2+ early-stage breast cancer receiving sequential anthracycline/trastuzumab, echocardiography-derived GLS was the most optimal prognostic marker even when compared to feature-tracking-derived GLS and global circumferential strain from CMR [72].

Given the inconclusive evidence to date, there is a need for further observational and randomized studies to determine the true potential of CMR in this setting.

6. Prevention and Treatment of CTRCD

As it has become evident that patients with cancer are at a heightened risk of developing cardiovascular disease. Given the existing knowledge in the pathophysiology and the presence of biomarkers for diagnosis and prognosis of CTRCD, research in the field is now focused on ways of preventing and treating CTRCD. In the field of prevention, several studies have been conducted. In patients diagnosed with cancer who had an indication to receive anthracycline chemotherapy, enalapril was tried as a preventive measure at the first chemotherapy cycle, while a control group received the medication at the time of troponin elevation during chemotherapy [73]. According to the results of this trial, the incidence of a troponin rise was similar across the two groups. Another study utilized the beta-blocker carvedilol in patients with HER2-negative breast cancer receiving anthracycline-containing treatment [74]. The authors found no differences in LVEF or troponin I levels between the carvedilol and placebo groups. The PRADA study compared multiple CTRCD prevention regimens in patients with early breast cancer [75]. At a median follow-up of 23 months, no differences in LVEF were noted in the studied groups (candesartan, metoprolol, placebo). Similarly, cardiac biomarkers (TnI, TnT, NTproBNP) were not significantly different with regards to treatment. Candesartan further failed to prevent cardiac events at a 2-year follow-up in 210 women with HER+ breast cancer who received anthracycline and trastuzumab as part of their chemotherapy [76]. It also did not affect cardiac biomarkers or the changes in LVEF compared to placebo. Among the promising agents in the prevention of CTRCD are mineralocorticoid receptor antagonists. Akpek et al., by utilizing a sample of 83 patients randomized to spironolactone or placebo, showed a significantly slower decline in LVEF with spironolactone, accompanied by steeper TnI rise and unaltered NTproBNP levels compared to placebo [77].

Treating CTRCD is another challenging task, often mandating the use of medications used for patients with HF. In the presence of mild, asymptomatic CTRCD that is indicated by abnormalities in GLS, TnI, or NTproBNP, the use of renin-angiotensin system blockers with or without beta-blockers is indicated by the existing European Society of Cardiology Cardio-oncology guidelines (Table 3) [3]. At least moderate and asymptomatic, or symptomatic CTRCD mandates the use of HF medications by following the related treatment algorithms [3]. For SGLT2 inhibitors in particular, Gongora et al. showed that the incidence of cardiac events (heart failure incidence-hospitalization, cardiotoxicity, clinically significant arrhythmias) was lower in diabetic patients receiving SGLT2 inhibitors compared to the control group [78]. A recent, larger-scale study compared the use of guideline-directed medical therapy with or without an SGLT2 inhibitor in patients with type 2 DM and CTRCD [79]. In a population of 6988 patients (654 used an SGLT2 inhibitor), the authors found a significantly lower incidence of all-cause mortality (OR: 0.296 [95% CI: 0.22–0.40]; $p = 0.001$) and HF decompensation (OR: 0.483 [95% CI: 0.36–0.65]; $p < 0.001$). Secondary endpoints were also favoring the use of SGLT2 inhibitors, namely the incidence of atrial fibrillation/flutter (OR: 0.397 [95% CI: 0.213–0.737]; $p = 0.003$), acute kidney injury (OR: 0.486 [95% CI: 0.382–0.619]; $p < 0.001$), and the need for renal replacement therapy (OR: 0.398 [95% CI: 0.189–0.839]; $p = 0.012$).

Table 3. Summary of the ESC guideline recommendations for the management of CTRCD associated with anthracyclines and anti-HER2 agents [3].

Symptomatic	CTRCD Severity	Recommendation (Class/Level)
AC		
Yes	Severe	HF therapy (I/B) Discontinue AC (I/C)
Yes	Moderate	HF therapy (I/B) Interrupt AC (I/C)
Yes	Mild	HF therapy (I/B) MDT for interruption vs. continuation (I/C)
No	Severe/Moderate	HF therapy (I/B) Interrupt AC (I/C)
No	Mild	Continue AC (I/C) ACEi/ARB and/or BB if GLS decreases/TnI increases (IIa/B) or NP increases (IIb/C)
Anti-HER2		
Yes	Severe/Moderate	HF therapy (I/B) Interrupt anti-HER2
Yes	Mild	HF therapy (I/B) MDT for interruption vs. continuation (I/C)
No	Severe	HF therapy (I/B) Interrupt anti-HER2
No	Moderate	Continue anti-HER2 (IIa/B) HF therapy (I/B)
No	Mild	Continue anti-HER2 (I/C) ACEi/ARB and/or BB if GLS decreases or TnI/NP increase (IIa/B)

AC: anthracycline, HF: heart failure, MDT: multidisciplinary team, ACEi: angiotensin-converting enzyme inhibitor, ARB: angiotensin receptor blocker, BB: beta blocker, GLS: global longitudinal strain, TnI: troponin I, and NP: natriuretic peptide.

7. Future Directions-Gaps in Evidence

Despite significant progress in the field of cardio-oncology, several critical gaps in knowledge and clinical practice remain. Early detection of CTRCD is a pressing challenge.

Current biomarkers, such as troponins and NT-proBNP, are reliable but often detect cardiac injury after irreversible dysfunction has occurred. Novel biomarkers, including galectin-3 and soluble ST2 (sST2), hold promise in identifying early myocardial stress or fibrosis but require further validation in large-scale clinical trials. Additionally, imaging modalities such as CMR and CT-derived extracellular volume measurements offer exciting potential for earlier detection of subclinical cardiac injury. However, studies are needed to define the optimal timing, cost-effectiveness, and real-world applicability of these advanced imaging tools.

Therapeutic innovations in CTRCD prevention also remain underexplored. While medications like spironolactone and SGLT2 inhibitors have shown potential in mitigating cardiac dysfunction, most evidence stems from small-scale studies. Multicenter, randomized controlled trials are urgently needed to confirm the effectiveness of these agents in broader populations. Similarly, while traditional cardioprotective agents such as beta-blockers and angiotensin-converting enzyme inhibitors are widely used, their role in specific high-risk subgroups or in combination with newer therapies has yet to be fully delineated. Investigating the interaction between cancer therapies and cardioprotective drugs, particularly in complex cases involving multiple comorbidities, should be prioritized to refine treatment protocols.

Personalized risk prediction and management represent another significant area for advancement. Current approaches to CTRCD prevention often rely on population-based strategies, which may overlook the heterogeneity of patient responses to cancer therapies. Developing precision medicine tools that integrate clinical, genetic, and treatment-specific factors can improve the prediction of CTRCD risk. Leveraging artificial intelligence and machine learning algorithms to analyze large datasets from clinical trials and registries could provide actionable insights for individualized management strategies. Such models could also help identify high-risk patients who would benefit most from intensive cardiac monitoring or early cardioprotective interventions.

Finally, fostering interdisciplinary collaboration and expanding access to cardio-oncology resources are essential to addressing gaps in care. Establishing international cardio-oncology registries could provide valuable real-world data on CTRCD incidence, treatment outcomes, and best practices. Additionally, efforts to adapt guidelines, such as those from the European Society of Cardiology (ESC), to diverse healthcare settings—including resource-limited environments—are critical for ensuring equitable care. Addressing implementation barriers, such as training for healthcare professionals and the financial burden of advanced diagnostic tools, will be crucial in optimizing outcomes for cancer patients globally. By addressing these challenges, future research and clinical efforts can ensure that advancements in cancer care are not achieved at the expense of cardiovascular health.

8. Conclusions

Cancer therapy-induced cardiotoxicity presents a growing concern as cancer survival rates improve. This adverse effect, particularly common with anthracyclines and targeted therapies like trastuzumab, underscores the need for a balance between effective cancer treatment and cardiovascular safety. Early detection using cardiac biomarkers and advanced imaging techniques, combined with preventive strategies like the use of beta-blockers or ACE inhibitors, can mitigate long-term cardiac damage. The evolution of cardio-oncology highlights the importance of an interdisciplinary approach, where collaboration between oncologists and cardiologists is key to reducing cardiovascular risks. As research advances, the development of targeted cardioprotective therapies offers promising avenues to safeguard patients' heart health without compromising cancer treatment efficacy. Ensuring continuous monitoring and personalized interventions will be crucial to improving both oncological and cardiovascular outcomes for cancer survivors.

Funding: This research received no external funding.

Conflicts of Interest: The authors declare no conflict of interest.

References

1. Stoltzfus, K.C.; Zhang, Y.; Sturgeon, K.; Sinoway, L.I.; Trifiletti, D.M.; Chinchilli, V.M.; Zaorsky, N.G. Fatal heart disease among cancer patients. *Nat. Commun.* **2020**, *11*, 2011. [CrossRef] [PubMed]
2. Suter, T.M.; Ewer, M.S. Cancer drugs and the heart: Importance and management. *Eur. Heart J.* **2013**, *34*, 1102–1111. [CrossRef]
3. Lyon, A.R.; Lopez-Fernandez, T.; Couch, L.S.; Asteggiano, R.; Aznar, M.C.; Bergler-Klein, J.; Boriani, G.; Cardinale, D.; Cordoba, R.; Cosyns, B.; et al. 2022 ESC Guidelines on cardio-oncology developed in collaboration with the European Hematology Association (EHA), the European Society for Therapeutic Radiology and Oncology (ESTRO) and the International Cardio-Oncology Society (IC-OS). *Eur. Heart J.* **2022**, *43*, 4229–4361. [CrossRef] [PubMed]
4. Herrmann, J.; Lenihan, D.; Armenian, S.; Barac, A.; Blaes, A.; Cardinale, D.; Carver, J.; Dent, S.; Ky, B.; Lyon, A.R.; et al. Defining cardiovascular toxicities of cancer therapies: An International Cardio-Oncology Society (IC-OS) consensus statement. *Eur. Heart J.* **2022**, *43*, 280–299. [CrossRef]
5. Wang, L.; Tan, T.C.; Halpern, E.F.; Neilan, T.G.; Francis, S.A.; Picard, M.H.; Fei, H.; Hochberg, E.P.; Abramson, J.S.; Weyman, A.E.; et al. Major Cardiac Events and the Value of Echocardiographic Evaluation in Patients Receiving Anthracycline-Based Chemotherapy. *Am. J. Cardiol.* **2015**, *116*, 442–446. [CrossRef] [PubMed]
6. Bostany, G.; Chen, Y.; Francisco, L.; Dai, C.; Meng, Q.; Sparks, J.; Sessions, M.; Nabell, L.; Stringer-Reasor, E.; Khoury, K.; et al. Cardiac Dysfunction Among Breast Cancer Survivors: Role of Cardiotoxic Therapy and Cardiovascular Risk Factors. *J. Clin. Oncol.* **2024**, JCO2301779. [CrossRef]
7. Limat, S.; Demesmay, K.; Voillat, L.; Bernard, Y.; Deconinck, E.; Brion, A.; Sabbah, A.; Woronoff-Lemsi, M.C.; Cahn, J.Y. Early cardiotoxicity of the CHOP regimen in aggressive non-Hodgkin's lymphoma. *Ann. Oncol.* **2003**, *14*, 277–281. [CrossRef] [PubMed]
8. Sawaya, H.; Sebag, I.A.; Plana, J.C.; Januzzi, J.L.; Ky, B.; Tan, T.C.; Cohen, V.; Banchs, J.; Carver, J.R.; Wiegers, S.E.; et al. Assessment of echocardiography and biomarkers for the extended prediction of cardiotoxicity in patients treated with anthracyclines, taxanes, and trastuzumab. *Circ. Cardiovasc. Imaging* **2012**, *5*, 596–603. [CrossRef]
9. Hundley, W.G.; D'Agostino, R., Jr.; Crotts, T.; Craver, K.; Hackney, M.H.; Jordan, J.H.; Ky, B.; Wagner, L.I.; Herrington, D.M.; Yeboah, J.; et al. Statins and Left Ventricular Ejection Fraction Following Doxorubicin Treatment. *NEJM Evid.* **2022**, *1*. [CrossRef] [PubMed]
10. Mulrooney, D.A.; Yeazel, M.W.; Kawashima, T.; Mertens, A.C.; Mitby, P.; Stovall, M.; Donaldson, S.S.; Green, D.M.; Sklar, C.A.; Robison, L.L.; et al. Cardiac outcomes in a cohort of adult survivors of childhood and adolescent cancer: Retrospective analysis of the Childhood Cancer Survivor Study cohort. *BMJ* **2009**, *339*, b4606. [CrossRef] [PubMed]
11. Armstrong, G.T.; Plana, J.C.; Zhang, N.; Srivastava, D.; Green, D.M.; Ness, K.K.; Daniel Donovan, F.; Metzger, M.L.; Arevalo, A.; Durand, J.B.; et al. Screening adult survivors of childhood cancer for cardiomyopathy: Comparison of echocardiography and cardiac magnetic resonance imaging. *J. Clin. Oncol.* **2012**, *30*, 2876–2884. [CrossRef]
12. Drafts, B.C.; Twomley, K.M.; D'Agostino, R., Jr.; Lawrence, J.; Avis, N.; Ellis, L.R.; Thohan, V.; Jordan, J.; Melin, S.A.; Torti, F.M.; et al. Low to moderate dose anthracycline-based chemotherapy is associated with early noninvasive imaging evidence of subclinical cardiovascular disease. *JACC Cardiovasc. Imaging* **2013**, *6*, 877–885. [CrossRef] [PubMed]
13. Greenlee, H.; Iribarren, C.; Rana, J.S.; Cheng, R.; Nguyen-Huynh, M.; Rillamas-Sun, E.; Shi, Z.; Laurent, C.A.; Lee, V.S.; Roh, J.M.; et al. Risk of Cardiovascular Disease in Women With and Without Breast Cancer: The Pathways Heart Study. *J. Clin. Oncol.* **2022**, *40*, 1647–1658. [CrossRef] [PubMed]
14. Henry, M.L.; Niu, J.; Zhang, N.; Giordano, S.H.; Chavez-MacGregor, M. Cardiotoxicity and Cardiac Monitoring Among Chemotherapy-Treated Breast Cancer Patients. *JACC Cardiovasc. Imaging* **2018**, *11*, 1084–1093. [CrossRef] [PubMed]
15. Bria, E.; Cuppone, F.; Fornier, M.; Nistico, C.; Carlini, P.; Milella, M.; Sperduti, I.; Terzoli, E.; Cognetti, F.; Giannarelli, D. Cardiotoxicity and incidence of brain metastases after adjuvant trastuzumab for early breast cancer: The dark side of the moon? A meta-analysis of the randomized trials. *Breast Cancer Res. Treat.* **2008**, *109*, 231–239. [CrossRef] [PubMed]
16. Slamon, D.; Eiermann, W.; Robert, N.; Pienkowski, T.; Martin, M.; Press, M.; Mackey, J.; Glaspy, J.; Chan, A.; Pawlicki, M.; et al. Adjuvant trastuzumab in HER2-positive breast cancer. *N. Engl. J. Med.* **2011**, *365*, 1273–1283. [CrossRef]
17. Gianni, L.; Eiermann, W.; Semiglazov, V.; Manikhas, A.; Lluch, A.; Tjulandin, S.; Zambetti, M.; Vazquez, F.; Byakhow, M.; Lichinitser, M.; et al. Neoadjuvant chemotherapy with trastuzumab followed by adjuvant trastuzumab versus neoadjuvant chemotherapy alone, in patients with HER2-positive locally advanced breast cancer (the NOAH trial): A randomised controlled superiority trial with a parallel HER2-negative cohort. *Lancet* **2010**, *375*, 377–384. [CrossRef] [PubMed]
18. Moja, L.; Tagliabue, L.; Balduzzi, S.; Parmelli, E.; Pistotti, V.; Guarneri, V.; D'Amico, R. Trastuzumab containing regimens for early breast cancer. *Cochrane Database Syst. Rev.* **2012**, *2012*, CD006243. [CrossRef]
19. Slamon, D.J.; Leyland-Jones, B.; Shak, S.; Fuchs, H.; Paton, V.; Bajamonde, A.; Fleming, T.; Eiermann, W.; Wolter, J.; Pegram, M.; et al. Use of chemotherapy plus a monoclonal antibody against HER2 for metastatic breast cancer that overexpresses HER2. *N. Engl. J. Med.* **2001**, *344*, 783–792. [CrossRef]
20. Seidman, A.; Hudis, C.; Pierri, M.K.; Shak, S.; Paton, V.; Ashby, M.; Murphy, M.; Stewart, S.J.; Keefe, D. Cardiac dysfunction in the trastuzumab clinical trials experience. *J. Clin. Oncol.* **2002**, *20*, 1215–1221. [CrossRef] [PubMed]
21. Shanmuganathan, J.W.D.; Kragholm, K.; Tayal, B.; Polcwiartek, C.; Poulsen, L.O.; El-Galaly, T.C.; Fosbol, E.L.; D'Souza, M.; Gislason, G.; Kober, L.; et al. Risk for Myocardial Infarction Following 5-Fluorouracil Treatment in Patients With Gastrointestinal Cancer: A Nationwide Registry-Based Study. *JACC CardioOncol.* **2021**, *3*, 725–733. [CrossRef]

22. Wacker, A.; Lersch, C.; Scherpinski, U.; Reindl, L.; Seyfarth, M. High incidence of angina pectoris in patients treated with 5-fluorouracil. A planned surveillance study with 102 patients. *Oncology* **2003**, *65*, 108–112. [CrossRef]
23. Jensen, S.A.; Hasbak, P.; Mortensen, J.; Sorensen, J.B. Fluorouracil induces myocardial ischemia with increases of plasma brain natriuretic peptide and lactic acid but without dysfunction of left ventricle. *J. Clin. Oncol.* **2010**, *28*, 5280–5286. [CrossRef] [PubMed]
24. Akhtar, S.S.; Salim, K.P.; Bano, Z.A. Symptomatic cardiotoxicity with high-dose 5-fluorouracil infusion: A prospective study. *Oncology* **1993**, *50*, 441–444. [CrossRef]
25. Shyam Sunder, S.; Sharma, U.C.; Pokharel, S. Adverse effects of tyrosine kinase inhibitors in cancer therapy: Pathophysiology, mechanisms and clinical management. *Signal Transduct. Target. Ther.* **2023**, *8*, 262. [CrossRef] [PubMed]
26. Ghatalia, P.; Morgan, C.J.; Je, Y.; Nguyen, P.L.; Trinh, Q.D.; Choueiri, T.K.; Sonpavde, G. Congestive heart failure with vascular endothelial growth factor receptor tyrosine kinase inhibitors. *Crit. Rev. Oncol. Hematol.* **2015**, *94*, 228–237. [CrossRef]
27. Herrmann, J.; Yang, E.H.; Iliescu, C.A.; Cilingiroglu, M.; Charitakis, K.; Hakeem, A.; Toutouzas, K.; Leesar, M.A.; Grines, C.L.; Marmagkiolis, K. Vascular Toxicities of Cancer Therapies: The Old and the New—An Evolving Avenue. *Circulation* **2016**, *133*, 1272–1289. [CrossRef]
28. Choi, H.D.; Chang, M.J. Cardiac toxicities of lapatinib in patients with breast cancer and other HER2-positive cancers: A meta-analysis. *Breast Cancer Res. Treat.* **2017**, *166*, 927–936. [CrossRef]
29. Dickerson, T.; Wiczer, T.; Waller, A.; Philippon, J.; Porter, K.; Haddad, D.; Guha, A.; Rogers, K.A.; Bhat, S.; Byrd, J.C.; et al. Hypertension and incident cardiovascular events following ibrutinib initiation. *Blood* **2019**, *134*, 1919–1928. [CrossRef] [PubMed]
30. Ghatalia, P.; Je, Y.; Kaymakcalan, M.D.; Sonpavde, G.; Choueiri, T.K. QTc interval prolongation with vascular endothelial growth factor receptor tyrosine kinase inhibitors. *Br. J. Cancer* **2015**, *112*, 296–305. [CrossRef]
31. Diaz-Serrano, A.; Gella, P.; Jimenez, E.; Zugazagoitia, J.; Paz-Ares Rodriguez, L. Targeting EGFR in Lung Cancer: Current Standards and Developments. *Drugs* **2018**, *78*, 893–911. [CrossRef]
32. Curigliano, G.; Lenihan, D.; Fradley, M.; Ganatra, S.; Barac, A.; Blaes, A.; Herrmann, J.; Porter, C.; Lyon, A.R.; Lancellotti, P.; et al. Management of cardiac disease in cancer patients throughout oncological treatment: ESMO consensus recommendations. *Ann. Oncol.* **2020**, *31*, 171–190. [CrossRef] [PubMed]
33. Mahmood, S.S.; Fradley, M.G.; Cohen, J.V.; Nohria, A.; Reynolds, K.L.; Heinzerling, L.M.; Sullivan, R.J.; Damrongwatanasuk, R.; Chen, C.L.; Gupta, D.; et al. Myocarditis in Patients Treated With Immune Checkpoint Inhibitors. *J. Am. Coll. Cardiol.* **2018**, *71*, 1755–1764. [CrossRef] [PubMed]
34. Cho, J.; Kim, H.S.; Ku, B.M.; Choi, Y.L.; Cristescu, R.; Han, J.; Sun, J.M.; Lee, S.H.; Ahn, J.S.; Park, K.; et al. Pembrolizumab for Patients With Refractory or Relapsed Thymic Epithelial Tumor: An Open-Label Phase II Trial. *J. Clin. Oncol.* **2019**, *37*, 2162–2170. [CrossRef] [PubMed]
35. Salem, J.E.; Manouchehri, A.; Moey, M.; Lebrun-Vignes, B.; Bastarache, L.; Pariente, A.; Gobert, A.; Spano, J.P.; Balko, J.M.; Bonaca, M.P.; et al. Cardiovascular toxicities associated with immune checkpoint inhibitors: An observational, retrospective, pharmacovigilance study. *Lancet Oncol.* **2018**, *19*, 1579–1589. [CrossRef]
36. Moslehi, J.J.; Salem, J.E.; Sosman, J.A.; Lebrun-Vignes, B.; Johnson, D.B. Increased reporting of fatal immune checkpoint inhibitor-associated myocarditis. *Lancet* **2018**, *391*, 933. [CrossRef] [PubMed]
37. Khunger, A.; Battel, L.; Wadhawan, A.; More, A.; Kapoor, A.; Agrawal, N. New Insights into Mechanisms of Immune Checkpoint Inhibitor-Induced Cardiovascular Toxicity. *Curr. Oncol. Rep.* **2020**, *22*, 65. [CrossRef]
38. Pohl, J.; Mincu, R.I.; Mrotzek, S.M.; Hinrichs, L.; Michel, L.; Livingstone, E.; Zimmer, L.; Wakili, R.; Schadendorf, D.; Rassaf, T.; et al. ECG Changes in Melanoma Patients Undergoing Cancer Therapy-Data From the ECoR Registry. *J. Clin. Med.* **2020**, *9*, 2060. [CrossRef] [PubMed]
39. Abdul-Rahman, T.; Dunham, A.; Huang, H.; Bukhari, S.M.A.; Mehta, A.; Awuah, W.A.; Ede-Imafidon, D.; Cantu-Herrera, E.; Talukder, S.; Joshi, A.; et al. Chemotherapy Induced Cardiotoxicity: A State of the Art Review on General Mechanisms, Prevention, Treatment and Recent Advances in Novel Therapeutics. *Curr. Probl. Cardiol.* **2023**, *48*, 101591. [CrossRef] [PubMed]
40. Angsutararux, P.; Luanpitpong, S.; Issaragrisil, S. Chemotherapy-Induced Cardiotoxicity: Overview of the Roles of Oxidative Stress. *Oxid. Med. Cell. Longev.* **2015**, *2015*, 795602. [CrossRef]
41. Ambrosio, G.; Zweier, J.L.; Duilio, C.; Kuppusamy, P.; Santoro, G.; Elia, P.P.; Tritto, I.; Cirillo, P.; Condorelli, M.; Chiariello, M.; et al. Evidence that mitochondrial respiration is a source of potentially toxic oxygen free radicals in intact rabbit hearts subjected to ischemia and reflow. *J. Biol. Chem.* **1993**, *268*, 18532–18541. [CrossRef]
42. Fariss, M.W.; Chan, C.B.; Patel, M.; Van Houten, B.; Orrenius, S. Role of mitochondria in toxic oxidative stress. *Mol. Interv.* **2005**, *5*, 94–111. [CrossRef] [PubMed]
43. Paradies, G.; Petrosillo, G.; Pistolese, M.; Di Venosa, N.; Federici, A.; Ruggiero, F.M. Decrease in mitochondrial complex I activity in ischemic/reperfused rat heart: Involvement of reactive oxygen species and cardiolipin. *Circ. Res.* **2004**, *94*, 53–59. [CrossRef]
44. Paradies, G.; Petrosillo, G.; Pistolese, M.; Ruggiero, F.M. The effect of reactive oxygen species generated from the mitochondrial electron transport chain on the cytochrome c oxidase activity and on the cardiolipin content in bovine heart submitochondrial particles. *FEBS Lett.* **2000**, *466*, 323–326. [CrossRef] [PubMed]
45. Lazzerini, P.E.; Capecchi, P.L.; Laghi-Pasini, F. Long QT Syndrome: An Emerging Role for Inflammation and Immunity. *Front. Cardiovasc. Med.* **2015**, *2*, 26. [CrossRef] [PubMed]

46. Aromolaran, A.S.; Srivastava, U.; Ali, A.; Chahine, M.; Lazaro, D.; El-Sherif, N.; Capecchi, P.L.; Laghi-Pasini, F.; Lazzerini, P.E.; Boutjdir, M. Interleukin-6 inhibition of hERG underlies risk for acquired long QT in cardiac and systemic inflammation. *PLoS ONE* **2018**, *13*, e0208321. [CrossRef] [PubMed]
47. Ali, A.; Boutjdir, M.; Aromolaran, A.S. Cardiolipotoxicity, Inflammation, and Arrhythmias: Role for Interleukin-6 Molecular Mechanisms. *Front. Physiol.* **2018**, *9*, 1866. [CrossRef]
48. Li, Q.; Qin, M.; Tan, Q.; Li, T.; Gu, Z.; Huang, P.; Ren, L. MicroRNA-129-1-3p protects cardiomyocytes from pirarubicin-induced apoptosis by down-regulating the GRIN2D-mediated Ca(2+) signalling pathway. *J. Cell. Mol. Med.* **2020**, *24*, 2260–2271. [CrossRef]
49. Sag, C.M.; Kohler, A.C.; Anderson, M.E.; Backs, J.; Maier, L.S. CaMKII-dependent SR Ca leak contributes to doxorubicin-induced impaired Ca handling in isolated cardiac myocytes. *J. Mol. Cell. Cardiol.* **2011**, *51*, 749–759. [CrossRef] [PubMed]
50. Sutanto, H.; Lyon, A.; Lumens, J.; Schotten, U.; Dobrev, D.; Heijman, J. Cardiomyocyte calcium handling in health and disease: Insights from in vitro and in silico studies. *Prog. Biophys. Mol. Biol.* **2020**, *157*, 54–75. [CrossRef]
51. Forstermann, U.; Munzel, T. Endothelial nitric oxide synthase in vascular disease: From marvel to menace. *Circulation* **2006**, *113*, 1708–1714. [CrossRef]
52. Taimeh, Z.; Loughran, J.; Birks, E.J.; Bolli, R. Vascular endothelial growth factor in heart failure. *Nat. Rev. Cardiol.* **2013**, *10*, 519–530. [CrossRef] [PubMed]
53. Shi, H.; Gao, Y.; Dong, Z.; Yang, J.; Gao, R.; Li, X.; Zhang, S.; Ma, L.; Sun, X.; Wang, Z.; et al. GSDMD-Mediated Cardiomyocyte Pyroptosis Promotes Myocardial I/R Injury. *Circ. Res.* **2021**, *129*, 383–396. [CrossRef] [PubMed]
54. Chintalgattu, V.; Ai, D.; Langley, R.R.; Zhang, J.; Bankson, J.A.; Shih, T.L.; Reddy, A.K.; Coombes, K.R.; Daher, I.N.; Pati, S.; et al. Cardiomyocyte PDGFR-beta signaling is an essential component of the mouse cardiac response to load-induced stress. *J. Clin. Investig.* **2010**, *120*, 472–484. [CrossRef] [PubMed]
55. Hagiwara, Y.; Miyoshi, S.; Fukuda, K.; Nishiyama, N.; Ikegami, Y.; Tanimoto, K.; Murata, M.; Takahashi, E.; Shimoda, K.; Hirano, T.; et al. SHP2-mediated signaling cascade through gp130 is essential for LIF-dependent I CaL, [Ca2+]i transient, and APD increase in cardiomyocytes. *J. Mol. Cell. Cardiol.* **2007**, *43*, 710–716. [CrossRef] [PubMed]
56. Villegas, S.; Villarreal, F.J.; Dillmann, W.H. Leukemia Inhibitory Factor and Interleukin-6 downregulate sarcoplasmic reticulum Ca2+ ATPase (SERCA2) in cardiac myocytes. *Basic Res. Cardiol.* **2000**, *95*, 47–54. [CrossRef] [PubMed]
57. Tanaka, T.; Kanda, T.; Takahashi, T.; Saegusa, S.; Moriya, J.; Kurabayashi, M. Interleukin-6-induced reciprocal expression of SERCA and natriuretic peptides mRNA in cultured rat ventricular myocytes. *J. Int. Med. Res.* **2004**, *32*, 57–61. [CrossRef]
58. Fontes, J.A.; Rose, N.R.; Cihakova, D. The varying faces of IL-6: From cardiac protection to cardiac failure. *Cytokine* **2015**, *74*, 62–68. [CrossRef]
59. Yamauchi-Takihara, K.; Kishimoto, T. Cytokines and their receptors in cardiovascular diseases—Role of gp130 signalling pathway in cardiac myocyte growth and maintenance. *Int. J. Exp. Pathol.* **2000**, *81*, 1–16. [CrossRef] [PubMed]
60. Feldman, A.M.; Combes, A.; Wagner, D.; Kadakomi, T.; Kubota, T.; Li, Y.Y.; McTiernan, C. The role of tumor necrosis factor in the pathophysiology of heart failure. *J. Am. Coll. Cardiol.* **2000**, *35*, 537–544. [CrossRef] [PubMed]
61. Cappetta, D.; Esposito, G.; Coppini, R.; Piegari, E.; Russo, R.; Ciuffreda, L.P.; Rivellino, A.; Santini, L.; Rafaniello, C.; Scavone, C.; et al. Effects of ranolazine in a model of doxorubicin-induced left ventricle diastolic dysfunction. *Br. J. Pharmacol.* **2017**, *174*, 3696–3712. [CrossRef]
62. Ponde, N.F.; Lambertini, M.; de Azambuja, E. Twenty years of anti-HER2 therapy-associated cardiotoxicity. *ESMO Open* **2016**, *1*, e000073. [CrossRef] [PubMed]
63. Xu, T.; Meng, Q.H.; Gilchrist, S.C.; Lin, S.H.; Lin, R.; Xu, T.; Milgrom, S.A.; Gandhi, S.J.; Wu, H.; Zhao, Y.; et al. Assessment of Prognostic Value of High-Sensitivity Cardiac Troponin T for Early Prediction of Chemoradiation Therapy-Induced Cardiotoxicity in Patients with Non-Small Cell Lung Cancer: A Secondary Analysis of a Prospective Randomized Trial. *Int. J. Radiat. Oncol. Biol. Phys.* **2021**, *111*, 907–916. [CrossRef]
64. Finke, D.; Romann, S.W.; Heckmann, M.B.; Hund, H.; Bougatf, N.; Kantharajah, A.; Katus, H.A.; Muller, O.J.; Frey, N.; Giannitsis, E.; et al. High-sensitivity cardiac troponin T determines all-cause mortality in cancer patients: A single-centre cohort study. *ESC Heart Fail.* **2021**, *8*, 3709–3719. [CrossRef] [PubMed]
65. Lv, X.; Pan, C.; Guo, H.; Chang, J.; Gao, X.; Wu, X.; Zhi, X.; Ren, C.; Chen, Q.; Jiang, H.; et al. Early diagnostic value of high-sensitivity cardiac troponin T for cancer treatment-related cardiac dysfunction: A meta-analysis. *ESC Heart Fail.* **2023**, *10*, 2170–2182. [CrossRef] [PubMed]
66. Liu, Y.; Zhang, T.; Huang, X.; Shen, L.; Yang, Q. Changes in Epicardial Adipose Tissue Assessed by Chest CT in Breast Cancer Patients Receiving Adjuvant Chemotherapy with Anthracyclines and Trastuzumab. *Rev. Cardiovasc. Med.* **2024**, *25*, 254. [CrossRef]
67. Rosenfeld, R.; Riondino, S.; Cerocchi, M.; Luciano, A.; Idone, G.; Lecis, D.; Illuminato, F.; Tolomei, A.; Torino, F.; Chiocchi, M.; et al. Extracellular volume measured by whole body CT scans predicts chronic cardiotoxicity in breast cancer patients treated with neoadjuvant therapies based on anthracyclines: A retrospective study. *Breast* **2024**, *76*, 103755. [CrossRef]
68. Lustberg, M.B.; Reinbolt, R.; Addison, D.; Ruppert, A.S.; Moore, S.; Carothers, S.; Suresh, A.; Das, H.; Berger, M.; Ramaswamy, B.; et al. Early Detection of Anthracycline-Induced Cardiotoxicity in Breast Cancer Survivors With T2 Cardiac Magnetic Resonance. *Circ. Cardiovasc. Imaging* **2019**, *12*, e008777. [CrossRef]
69. Thavendiranathan, P.; Shalmon, T.; Fan, C.S.; Houbois, C.; Amir, E.; Thevakumaran, Y.; Somerset, E.; Malowany, J.M.; Urzua-Fresno, C.; Yip, P.; et al. Comprehensive Cardiovascular Magnetic Resonance Tissue Characterization and Cardiotoxicity in Women With Breast Cancer. *JAMA Cardiol.* **2023**, *8*, 524–534. [CrossRef] [PubMed]

70. Buck, B.; Chum, A.P.; Patel, M.; Carter, R.; Nawaz, H.; Yildiz, V.; Ruz, P.; Wiczer, T.; Rogers, K.A.; Awan, F.T.; et al. Cardiovascular Magnetic Resonance Imaging in Patients With Ibrutinib-Associated Cardiotoxicity. *JAMA Oncol.* **2023**, *9*, 552–555. [CrossRef]
71. van Woerden, G.; van Veldhuisen, D.J.; Manintveld, O.C.; van Empel, V.P.M.; Willems, T.P.; de Boer, R.A.; Rienstra, M.; Westenbrink, B.D.; Gorter, T.M. Epicardial Adipose Tissue and Outcome in Heart Failure With Mid-Range and Preserved Ejection Fraction. *Circ. Heart Fail.* **2022**, *15*, e009238. [CrossRef] [PubMed]
72. Houbois, C.P.; Nolan, M.; Somerset, E.; Shalmon, T.; Esmaeilzadeh, M.; Lamacie, M.M.; Amir, E.; Brezden-Masley, C.; Koch, C.A.; Thevakumaran, Y.; et al. Serial Cardiovascular Magnetic Resonance Strain Measurements to Identify Cardiotoxicity in Breast Cancer: Comparison With Echocardiography. *JACC Cardiovasc. Imaging* **2021**, *14*, 962–974. [CrossRef] [PubMed]
73. Cardinale, D.; Ciceri, F.; Latini, R.; Franzosi, M.G.; Sandri, M.T.; Civelli, M.; Cucchi, G.; Menatti, E.; Mangiavacchi, M.; Cavina, R.; et al. Anthracycline-induced cardiotoxicity: A multicenter randomised trial comparing two strategies for guiding prevention with enalapril: The International CardioOncology Society-one trial. *Eur. J. Cancer* **2018**, *94*, 126–137. [CrossRef]
74. Avila, M.S.; Ayub-Ferreira, S.M.; de Barros Wanderley, M.R., Jr.; das Dores Cruz, F.; Goncalves Brandao, S.M.; Rigaud, V.O.C.; Higuchi-Dos-Santos, M.H.; Hajjar, L.A.; Kalil Filho, R.; Hoff, P.M.; et al. Carvedilol for Prevention of Chemotherapy-Related Cardiotoxicity: The CECCY Trial. *J. Am. Coll. Cardiol.* **2018**, *71*, 2281–2290. [CrossRef] [PubMed]
75. Heck, S.L.; Mecinaj, A.; Ree, A.H.; Hoffmann, P.; Schulz-Menger, J.; Fagerland, M.W.; Gravdehaug, B.; Rosjo, H.; Steine, K.; Geisler, J.; et al. Prevention of Cardiac Dysfunction During Adjuvant Breast Cancer Therapy (PRADA): Extended Follow-Up of a 2x2 Factorial, Randomized, Placebo-Controlled, Double-Blind Clinical Trial of Candesartan and Metoprolol. *Circulation* **2021**, *143*, 2431–2440. [CrossRef]
76. Boekhout, A.H.; Gietema, J.A.; Milojkovic Kerklaan, B.; van Werkhoven, E.D.; Altena, R.; Honkoop, A.; Los, M.; Smit, W.M.; Nieboer, P.; Smorenburg, C.H.; et al. Angiotensin II-Receptor Inhibition With Candesartan to Prevent Trastuzumab-Related Cardiotoxic Effects in Patients With Early Breast Cancer: A Randomized Clinical Trial. *JAMA Oncol.* **2016**, *2*, 1030–1037. [CrossRef] [PubMed]
77. Akpek, M.; Ozdogru, I.; Sahin, O.; Inanc, M.; Dogan, A.; Yazici, C.; Berk, V.; Karaca, H.; Kalay, N.; Oguzhan, A.; et al. Protective effects of spironolactone against anthracycline-induced cardiomyopathy. *Eur. J. Heart Fail.* **2015**, *17*, 81–89. [CrossRef] [PubMed]
78. Gongora, C.A.; Drobni, Z.D.; Quinaglia Araujo Costa Silva, T.; Zafar, A.; Gong, J.; Zlotoff, D.A.; Gilman, H.K.; Hartmann, S.E.; Sama, S.; Nikolaidou, S.; et al. Sodium-Glucose Co-Transporter-2 Inhibitors and Cardiac Outcomes Among Patients Treated With Anthracyclines. *JACC Heart Fail.* **2022**, *10*, 559–567. [CrossRef]
79. Avula, V.; Sharma, G.; Kosiborod, M.N.; Vaduganathan, M.; Neilan, T.G.; Lopez, T.; Dent, S.; Baldassarre, L.; Scherrer-Crosbie, M.; Barac, A.; et al. SGLT2 Inhibitor Use and Risk of Clinical Events in Patients With Cancer Therapy-Related Cardiac Dysfunction. *JACC Heart Fail.* **2024**, *12*, 67–78. [CrossRef]

MDPI AG
Grosspeteranlage 5
4052 Basel
Switzerland
Tel.: +41 61 683 77 34

Biomedicines Editorial Office
E-mail: biomedicines@mdpi.com
www.mdpi.com/journal/biomedicines